Dedication

For Paul and Sue, who taught me that an unlocked door, in and of itself, is not a bad thing.

E.A.M.

Table of Contents

Table of Contents

ONE

Not My Turn

"Not my turn," she answered her mother, brushing her blond hair away from her face. "I did it last, r-remember?" Standing on a chair in the kitchen, Elizabeth continued drying the stack of dinner plates and returning them to their rightful place in the cupboard.

Mom's pear-shaped frame, the result of birthing seven children and enduring nine miscarriages, turned from the oven. Looking at her daughter in annoyance and distrust, she turned toward the kitchen archway. "Emma! *Emmma!*"

Elizabeth's eleven-year-old sister, Emma, entered the kitchen, a plastic Barbie's platinum-blonde head poking out from beneath her armpit.

"Your father has a headache," Mom said. "Guess it's your turn." Mom turned back toward the stove.

1

Emma paused. "I think it's Sarah's turn."

Mom sighed.

"Really, it's Sarah's turn," Emma pled. "Remember? I missed church on Wednesday. Dad had a headache, and I had to stay home."

This truth could not be denied, and another bellow sounded from the kitchen.

"Sarah! Sarah!" Mom belted out as Elizabeth and Emma locked eyes. Elizabeth's heart pounded as she waited for her nine-year-old sister to appear. In a moment, Sarah's freckled face poked around the doorway.

"Yeah, Mom?" she asked, stepping over the kitchen threshold.

"Your father has a headache," Mom said, now slicing celery on the countertop. "Your sisters say it's your turn."

"Um, no," Sarah replied, furrowing her brow. "I think I went last—"

Slamming the knife onto the kitchen counter, their mother turned around. "God!" she shrilled. "Your father works double shifts for this family, and you can't even rub his neck when he gets migraines?"

Silence enveloped the kitchen. Elizabeth and her sisters stood motionless, unblinking, barely breathing, unwilling to draw the least bit of attention.

"Wait a minute," Mom replied, enunciating the *t*'s through clenched teeth. "What kind of mother am I if I can't make my own children obey?" Facing Elizabeth, Mom raised her eyebrows. "I asked you first, and you will obey. Maybe you should do a little more Bible reading. Ephesians six, perhaps?"

Still holding the dish towel, Elizabeth dared not reply. Nor did she obey.

"I said go," Mom threatened, taking a menacing step toward her.

Elizabeth jumped down from her chair, dropped the dish towel on the counter, and hurried past her sisters. Stopping at the base of the brown staircase that led to her father's bedroom, she turned toward the kitchen and tried to speak several times, but her throat was constricted. "M-m-mom," she stammered at last.

"Dear Jesus, *what?*" Mom yelled.

"W-w-when will m-my turn b-be over?"

"The sooner you get started, the sooner you'll be done," Mom decreed.

Turning back toward the staircase, Elizabeth rested her bare foot on the first step. A familiar dullness crept over her brain.

As she closed her eyes and ascended the steps, the humming began in her head, the white noise that washed over her in a steady crescendo, encompassing her.

She reached the top step, and her eyes mechanically opened. She turned left. Through the open door of her father's bedroom, she recognized the familiar shape of his naked body beneath the sheets.

She entered his bedroom and nodded to the raised, white, swirled paint covering the walls and ceiling, and they leaped to her in greeting. Rubbing her thumb and index finger together, her skin transformed into crisp, grooved ridges.

Transfixed at the foot of his mattress, she read the neon red digits of the clock on the nightstand: 1:00.

"Hi Lizzie," Dad mumbled, glancing at her, then turning away, burying his face in the crook of his elbow.

Climbing up onto the mattress, she positioned herself next to him, on her knees. She began rubbing his neck. Tilting her face upward to avoid his scent of oil, grease, and body odor, she knew his breath would smell like coffee. As she massaged his neck, he moaned in appreciation.

Moments passed. He shook his shoulders, and at that signal, she slid her hands down his pale, freckled back and began kneading his torso.

Looking at the clock, she smiled at the red digits: 1:30. Her turn was already half over.

He shook his shoulders again.

Compliant, she scooted back, preparing to lie down on her side.

Dad rolled from his stomach onto his back, and the white pillow now cradled his head. Raising his left forearm, he shielded his eyes from the light.

Easing onto her left side, she awaited his direction. He reached for her right hand and drew it to his chest, moving her palm in a soft, circular, rubbing motion. His nipples sprang upward, hardening like tiny pieces of rubber.

Eyeing the clock, she saw it was 1:59. At the crucial minute, the call from her mother did not come. Elizabeth sighed. Today her shift would be two hours long.

TWO

H o p e

My therapist qualification requirements were threefold:

One, she must not be a Christian…or at least must not market herself as one. My parents were Christians, so I'm not going there.

Two, she must be a woman. Men cause me to feel confused and overwhelmed. I'm not paying money to any man.

Three, she must accept my current insurance provider. My insurance company gave me the names of three therapists, and one was a woman. That simplified matters.

Inside the Mental Health Professionals lobby, pretending to read a magazine, I scan the room disconcertedly. It's not that I'm reluctant to be here. After all, I made a promise to my husband, and I'm keeping it.

Shifting in my seat and crossing my legs, I resist the urge to leave, even as I contemplate this concept of "therapy" and its purported idyllic benefits. How can talking to someone in an enclosed room help me or, for that matter, help anyone?

Seeking counsel from a total stranger could be considered unwise, but for me, it's at least *wiser.* I've never demonstrated good judgment, and anyone who knows me would probably describe me as weak. Trusting a stranger to help me deal with life may be a crap shoot, but it's certainly less risky than trusting myself. I already know not to do that. On my own, I've nearly destroyed the only relationship I've ever cared about.

The waiting-room door opens, revealing a small woman wearing leather sandals, gray slacks, and a blue cotton sweater. Her large blue-gray eyes offer a refined, astute appearance. My father would have disapproved of her brown hair, cut short, and asked her if she knew whether she was a girl or a boy.

"Elizabeth?" she softly inquires.

I rise from my chair, and the lady waits as I cross the room. Then she closes the door behind me and extends her hand.

"My name's Maureen McNamara. Nice to meet you," she says.

Smiling, I return her handshake, not speaking for fear I'll stutter.

She ushers me down a short hall to a large oak door. Removing a key from her pocket, she opens the door, and we enter a small office with a view of the early spring budding dogwoods. Closing this door, she extends her hand again, this time toward a pink, soft-looking cottony chair to my right. The room, lit only by the midday sun, provides a blanketed, calm feeling, as if I have entered a cocoon.

I sit, and she takes a seat across from me. I take a big breath and think, *here we go.*

She smiles with her eyes now. "What brings you here today, Elizabeth? Do you go by Elizabeth?"

"L-Liz," I say, wincing as I stutter on the first word.

"Liz, then. What brings you here?"

"I made an agreement with my husband, Matt. I told him if I used my white wall again, I'd get counseling. So here I am." I clear my throat. "So I'm here, honoring my agreement," I add.

"Okay," she begins. "You and Matt—your husband—made an agreement?"

I nod.

"And you said something about a white wall?"

I nod again.

"When I'm upset, I g-go to my white wall. Matt says its weird." I pause, aware my voice is now trembling. "Anyway, w-we agreed if I used it again, I'd get c-counseling. We had a fight last week, and I tried not to use it, b-but I had to." I wonder if she thinks my white wall is weird. I wonder if she is already tired of my stuttering.

"Liz, how are you feeling?" she asks.

My initial hesitation, waning at her surprisingly courteous, almost kind question takes me by surprise. I realize I have been holding my breath.

"F-fragile," I whisper as I exhale. "Like I can't handle anything. Like I will break into a million pieces any second."

"Can you tell me what you are most afraid of?"

"That M-Matt will leave me." My voice cracks. "Without him I will die." Covering my face with my hands and taking in a slow, deep breath, I attempt to compose myself.

Maureen waits. "You're afraid Matt will leave you?"

Nodding, I reach for a tissue.

"It could be helpful to explore your relationship with Matt. And it will be important to learn how to take care of you, *yourself,* emotionally."

I wonder what taking care of myself emotionally looks like and what it feels like.

"Liz, can you tell me about yourself? Anything that troubles you now or troubled you growing up?"

"When I was a kid, my dad went to jail for the back rubs. The judge who sentenced him was a worldly judge, not from our church. He never understood what happened, how Dad had migraines and needed the back rubs to keep his mind off the pain."

"Maybe you can help me understand," Maureen says.

Maureen wasn't from our church, so I didn't expect her to understand. But I could tell she *wanted* to understand.

"Dad had migraines and needed back rubs to keep his mind off the pain. Mom had a schedule for us three older girls and sent us up one at a time, usually for a one-hour shift, but sometimes two hours, depending. When your turn was over, Mom would call you down and send the next one up."

"When you say 'back rubs,' do you mean you rubbed his back?"

"Yes, sort of. His neck first," I begin. "Then his back, his front, and then, his legs, and…then, his private area…" My voice trailed off. "Sometimes he'd touch me, but we never had sex, not that I remember. Not like Matt and I have sex. The touching was to keep his mind off the pain, like I said."

I had never told the secret so plainly before. And then I realized I'd never told the secret at all.

"How often did this happen?"

Closing my eyes, I think. "I don't know if I can say an actual number. It was more than I washed the kitchen floor, which was every other week, but less than I did the dishes—that was every day. On average, I'd say once a week."

I await her verdict: am I attention seeking? Unstable? Mentally ill?

"Liz," Maureen says, folding her hands and placing them in her lap. "I'm so sorry that happened to you. It wasn't your fault."

In my silence I try to make sure I heard her correctly. I wait for her to add something, like a dirty face or ask me why I didn't stop it.

"It was not your fault," she repeats.

An enormous burden lifts from my shoulders, and I pause to bask in this great, warm quilt of words. A deep, penetrating warmth consumes my body, a body I realize might have been shivering for years. She has offered me the unexpected: genuine, simple, unmasked regret.

"I'm not c-crazy?" I whisper hopefully.

"Definitely not crazy," she replies with such certainty and sincerity, I can do nothing but believe her. She is, after all, a mental professional. She would know crazy if she saw it.

* * *

Home now, reveling in my newfound blamelessness, I pull out my journal and write, *It's not your fault*, and underline it. Then I write, *Definitely not crazy*, and underline it. I'm ready now. When the burden comes back to crush me, I'll reread this journal entry and remember I'm capable of feeling unaccountable, because I am feeling it today, March 29, 1989.

THREE

My Turn

Preparing for the final hour in Dad's bed, Elizabeth again tilted her head upward toward the ceiling. The white swirls called to her through the humming noise, and joining them, she traversed across the ceiling, easing to a stop as she blended into the sun-drenched, paint-chipped windowsill. Resting upon the ledge, she took comfort as the sun warmed her back.

He shook his shoulders again, and she moved her right hand down to his abdomen, continuing the circular motion. His jaw tightened, and she realized he knew she was stalling.

Grabbing her hand and forcing it beneath the sheets, he folded her four fingers around his penis until her index finger met her thumb. Placing his great hand around hers he squeezed her small fist, forming a tighter grip around his penis. As she began the familiar up-and-down motion, he splayed his legs, gradually releasing her hand, once satisfied with her rhythm.

Suddenly cold, she realized the sun had retreated behind a cloud. A white swirl caught her eye and she gave chase, again traveling up and across the ceiling, back down the wall, this time resting upon the wooden, paint-chipped floor.

Mechanically smiling a little girl's smile, she knew he would be pleased as he peeked at her.

"If I didn't have you, Lizzie, I would die," he confided. "The pain is too much for me to bear."

She turned the words over and over in her mind, comforted. He worked so hard for his family, double shifts even. He was one of the preachers at their church, and everybody loved him. Besides, she was his favorite daughter. He had told her so himself.

His breathing quickened and removing her hand from his penis, he turned toward her, pulling her close. His calloused palm was suddenly beneath her shirt. Her interrupted mind screamed to itself as he groped beneath her bra with the pink flower in the middle. Stomach churning and holding her breath, she waited for the pain. Her left nipple was scabbed over, and as his hand brushed her wounded breast, she inwardly flinched. He briefly hesitated before his rough fingers traveled the short distance to her small right breast.

The stench of coffee overpowered her as his bristly face tore at her cheeks and neck like sandpaper.

She blinked, and the humming crescendo reached the heavenly volume of ten thousand hummingbirds beating their wings in unison. Behind her eyelids, the white swirls formed at a prolific rate, cascading down her entire body. Her right hand floated upward toward her face and rested upon the raised, brittle ridges of her cheek. Bathed in iridescent whiteness, her transcendence complete, she was finally safe. And in the humming whiteness of it all, she felt nothing.

FOUR

The Deal

As the late morning sun filters across the page, I reread my journal entry again and toy with the idea that I am cured and needn't continue counseling. I look up at Matt as he prepares his lunch, his olive skin already tanned even though it is only the beginning of April. He is wearing his Sears repair uniform: navy blue pants and a dark blue short-sleeved shirt.

"You have to agree, Matt, I'm doing much better," I begin. "We could save some money if—"

"I agree you're doing better," he says, flashing his white smile. "And the deal is, we agreed on six months, and it's only been a week. Remember, I'm working until six tonight, so I'll be home a little late."

"Lawn mower season?" I ask.

"Job security season." He grins. "How late are you working?"

"Just until four, then I see Maureen." I say no more about skipping therapy. Tossing my journal and a pen into my work bag, today I plan to take notes during the session. Maybe by taking notes, I can get better faster.

I arrive on the children's unit at the psychiatric hospital. After keying myself in, I grab my sunscreen and sunglasses, then toss my bag into my locker. It's Wednesday and we always take the kids to the zoo on Wednesdays. My shift flies by, and after hugging the children good-bye, I head for Maureen's office. The drive is short, maybe five minutes, and along the way I smile at Matt's diplomacy. In three months we'll celebrate our first year of marriage, and I'm wondering if I'll be cured by then and what *cured* will feel like.

I smile in anticipation as Maureen unlocks her office door.

"How are you doing, Liz?" she asks, smiling as I sit down.

I realize she is not just being polite. "Fine, better," I say, holding up my pen and notebook. "I thought I'd take some notes."

She is still smiling as she reaches for a yellow tablet. "Do you mind if I take some notes, too?"

I hesitate. Secretaries transcribe and read patient notes, at least they do at the psychiatric hospital where I work. I don't want anyone reading about me. And what if I don't like what she writes about me? Would she ever give her notes to my parents? Surely she couldn't be working for them! Besides, why would she need to take notes? She's not the one who wants to get better.

I realize she has been awaiting my response.

"Who sees the notes?" I ask tentatively.

"No one except me; I use them to keep my information straight, to help me get to know you."

I realize for the first time I am not her only client. "Not your secretaries? Don't they transcribe?"

"No one transcribes here, Liz. Just two people will see them, you and me. I'll always give you a copy of what I write. See? I use carbon paper." She writes the date down then lifts the first yellow sheet, revealing the duplicate date beneath her original.

"What do you do with the notes after I leave?"

Rising, she takes three steps toward her desk. After pulling a small set of keys from her pocket, she unlocks a drawer with a tarnished knob, revealing an accordion-length stretch of file folders. "I keep them in here."

"No one else has a key?"

"No one," she confirms, locking her desk and sitting back down.

"And I always get a copy?" I ask.

"Always."

Less guarded, I choose to take what seems like a small risk. "Okay, then," I reply. "Okay."

Maureen's pen is poised, and I remind myself I can trust her.

"I was wondering," I begin. "Is there a way to feel how I felt last week? I mean, all the time. Not only right after I see you."

"What were you feeling last week?"

"Secure. And I'm more fluent. I ordered a hamburger through a drive-through and didn't stutter. I'm sleeping better, sometimes for the whole night. I don't remember the last time I slept through a whole night. But it's a fragile kind of secure. I mean, it could potentially fall apart at any moment."

"Feeling secure is important, Liz. We can look at that in a practical way. After all, nobody feels secure every single minute of every day. Perhaps being able to take care of yourself when you're scared? Is that a good place to start?"

Nodding, I'm relieved to hear nobody feels secure every minute of every day. I write down my first goal: *Take care of self when scared.*

"I want to get strong, like Matt, so when we fight he doesn't get so disgusted with me. That last argument, when I went to my white wall"—I pause—"he's never looked at me like that before."

"Can we talk about that argument?" she asks.

"Yeah, we were arguing about whose turn it was to fix dinner. I'm not like his mom that way—I don't want to work all day and then be expected to do everything at home, too, like laundry and meals. I love his mom, don't get me wrong, but we talked about this before we got married, how we'd share the house chores. Anyway, before I knew it, I was crying and on my way to my white wall. I mean I was trying hard not to go to my white wall, because I knew if I did, I'd have to see a counselor—that was our agreement. But I thought I was going to literally lose my mind. And if I went crazy? I'd lose him for sure. I *had* to go to my white wall."

"Did the argument end there?"

"Sort of. I mean, I woke up from my wall around one thirty in the morning. I climbed into bed, and he put his arm around me."

Maureen smiles.

"Yes, that was a relief. And then I asked if he still loved me, and he said yes. Then I asked him to *promise* he loved me."

"Did he?" she asks.

"Yes. Then I asked him to promise he doesn't think I'm used goods, and he doesn't think I'm a slut, and he promised."

Maureen looks up from her tablet and peers at me. "He promised you he didn't think you were used goods, and that you weren't a slut. You asked him to say that?"

"I ask him to say that after every argument."

"So after an argument, you ask him to promise he loves you and that you're not used goods and not a slut."

"Yes."

"And you do this because…"

I hesitate.

"How is that helpful to you?" she prompts.

"I've never thought about why."

Maureen is quiet, and I realize she's giving me time to think. Closing my eyes, I try to figure out the answer to her question.

"I guess I worry he looks down on me because of my family? We went to school in a small town, so I know people talked. I've told him little about my past."

"Does he know your father went to jail for sexually abusing you and your sisters?"

"Um, no. We moved to Bellevue after I got out of foster care, and although Dad was still in jail then, I just told people my parents were divorced. Sexual abuse isn't attractive," I add weakly. "I know I was dishonest; a lie of omission I guess is what I'd call it. And there've been times I've wondered if God will punish me with a divorce because I didn't tell Matt the whole truth. Maybe that's why we're having these problems now."

"So you think God might punish you?"

"Yes," I say, wondering if Maureen is Catholic. Just in case she is, I say a prayer for her in hopes she won't go to hell.

"Wait," I interject. "God doesn't believe in divorce, so He wouldn't do that. That'd make Him inconsistent. He'd pick something else."

"Have you ever wondered if God might understand why you didn't tell Matt the whole truth?"

I am reminded of my Aunt Sheila's God. "He might," I begin. "I mean, He could. It would be a big relief if He would do that." I jot this down in my journal as a prayer request.

"Okay. So Matt said he loved you; you weren't a slut; and you weren't used goods. Was the fight over?"

"Yes, except then he reminded me I agreed to get counseling."

She puts her pen down. "Do you think Matt is worried about you?"

"Yes," I reply, finding some solace in her words. "But I'm afraid I'm using up all of his concern. He didn't willingly sign up for this."

"We could invite Matt to one of our sessions," Maureen offers.

I look at her in surprise.

"We don't have to make a decision now, but if you want to include him and let him know what you're working through, we can. Of course if you don't want to, that's also fine. Doin' okay still?" she asks.

I nod.

"Good. Then let's change gears a bit. I know very little about your white wall. Could you tell me more about it?"

Pausing, I realize I've never explained my white wall to anyone, not even myself.

"My white wall has been a part of me for as long as I can remember," I begin slowly. "As a child, in high school, in college—it's always been a part of me. Since I've been on my own, whenever I move, I go to where my bedroom will be and find a wall. I spackle in any holes and repaint the wall white so it's ready when I need it. Then, when I get upset, I lie down on the floor in front of my wall. I don't really *look* at the wall," I say, squinting in concentration. "I go into it. I can feel the temperature of the wall and the paint texture on my skin. The wall and I become one. I feel tucked in, safe. When I need it, it's automatic. I blink a few times, the humming noise begins, and I'm in. And then when I'm feeling better, it turns off by itself, and it's like I'm whole again. I tried to give it up this last time, but it was as if my mind was going to break."

"The wall is a comfort to you," Maureen replies.

As I nod, I want to ask her again if she thinks I'm crazy. I wonder if there is a limit to how many times I can ask her this before she changes her mind.

"Liz, on Matt's behalf, your white wall may appear weird to someone raised in a normal family, and I use the word *normal* loosely," she qualifies. "But for someone with your particular life experience, the wall might be of benefit. If it helps you become peaceful, go for it. It's a childhood skill to be able to pull away. A time may come when you choose not to use your white wall, but now is not that time."

"Could you tell Matt that?" I ask hopefully.

"Maybe we could tell him together?" Maureen offers.

I smile in confirmation.

An alliance has been formed.

FIVE

Shift Change

The red digits revealed exactly three o'clock, and she held her breath, awaiting the voice of her salvation. Seconds stomped by as all around her time came and passed in whispered pleas.

At 3:01 her mind raced forward and backward. Was her mother punishing her? Was God punishing her? Did her mother forget about her?

A voice flying up the staircase grabbed her ears like a Christmas carol.

"Elizabeth?"

Mom!

"Your turn's up. How's his headache?"

Standing upright alongside his mattress, she bent down.

"How's your headache?" she whispered in his ear.

"Tell your mother to send up Emma with another pill," Dad moaned, palming his forehead with his right hand.

"Okay," she whispered. His smell saturated her hands, and she held them far out in front of her, away from her face.

"Well?" her mother asked as Elizabeth reached the bottom of the steps, then stopped.

"B-bad," she stammered, glancing briefly toward her mother. "He said send up Emma with another p-pill."

Her mother sighed. "Okay, go tell Emma to meet me in the kitchen. She's on the back porch."

Nodding, hands still extended, Elizabeth made her way toward the back porch in search of Emma. Glancing out the open back door, she saw her sitting on the concrete porch petting their cat, Smokey.

"Em, Mom wants you in the kitchen."

"Why?" asked Emma.

"D-dad's headache, it's your t-turn," answered Elizabeth.

"Already?" she groaned. "How long was your turn?"

"T-two hours," said Elizabeth. "Mom said now—"

"I'm going! Don't boss me!"

Now making her way toward the bathroom, Elizabeth closed the door and grabbed the slippery bar of soap. After lathering her arms up to her short shirt-sleeves, she washed her neck and face. Rinsing with warm water she reached for the hand towel and dried herself. Sniffing her arms, she frowned.

She could still smell him as she overheard Emma asking Mom when her shift would be over.

Lathering her hands again, she soaped up her arms then dug her nails into the bar, pressing the frothy lather into her nail beds.

After rinsing and drying herself again, she inhaled, furrowing her brow as the scent still lingered.

Where was it hiding?

She overheard her mother remind Emma to take a glass of water with her.

In her quiet panic, she took off her shirt, threw it to the floor, and reached for the soap a third time.

Vigorously lathering the bar, she rewashed her arms and face, and then her neck, taking care to cleanse her nostrils. She rinsed with warm water but didn't use the towel in case his smell had transferred there.

Opening the mirrored medicine cabinet, she reached for the rubbing alcohol and unscrewed the top. Dousing her hands, she quickly rubbed her palms together then slathered her face, neck, arms, and stomach with the medicinal liquid. Stooping down and grabbing her shirt, she ran her fingers through it, inside and out. Once she had her shirt back on, she filled her left palm with more rubbing alcohol, rubbed both hands together then patted her shirt on the front, sides, and shoulders.

Her eyes watering, she replaced the rubbing alcohol bottle cap. Trepidation coursing through her, she dared raise her palms to her face. Taking in short, shallow breaths, she was encouraged by the medicinal odor; she turned her hands over, sniffing her finger-nails. Her breathing slowed, and she tested her forearms and the tops of her shoulders. His scent was gone.

She looked in the mirror and smiled.

SIX

My Parents

Today Maureen asks me to tell her about my parents.

Dad and Mom divorced about two years ago and have each remarried. Dad married his brother's ex-wife, Florence. Mom married a guy named Ted.

"Poor Ted," I say. "If he only knew the kind of person Mom really was, he'd run screaming. I haven't seen Mom in over two years and don't miss her at all. If she died, I might attend her funeral but just to make sure she was really dead.

"Now, Dad? I see him pretty regularly—holidays and birthdays. As a kid I was always his favorite, and I'm still his favorite. Growing up, Dad was the nice parent. At the lake he'd be the alligator and all six of us kids were the fish. He'd come creeping up the bank, snorting and roaring and try to snatch us. When he caught one

24

of us, he'd take us out to sea then dunk us, transforming us into helper alligators. Then together we'd slink back to the shore and go after another fish.

"And when I was named Student of the Month at my high school, Dad carried around the newspaper clipping of me in his wallet. He'd take it out and show it to people and say, 'Hey, let me show you my kid.'"

"He was proud of you," Maureen says.

"He was. And when he had work to do, like cutting wood? We *all* worked, Dad included. But Mom? She was the opposite. She *assigned* work, especially to me and Emma. And while we worked? She'd read a book or watch a soap opera.

"Dad's the one who hugged and kissed us. I don't remember Mom hugging me unless we were at church, and she was putting on a show for people. I remember her touch always felt awkward, foreign."

"And Dad *never* called us upstairs for the back rubs. Mom arranged all that. If she got mad at you, she'd give you two shifts in a row. Double duty, she called it." My voice quivers in the throes of this memory. "Sometimes she'd change the rotation so if you went last, you'd still have to go first the next time. There was no way to prepare myself for my turn, because she was always switching it up." I feel the hairs on the back of my neck raise up.

"I know she hated having sex with Dad, but she could have taken a turn herself—then I'd only had to go every fourth time instead of every third time."

"She didn't like having sex with your dad?"

"You'd never know it with all the kids she had, but yeah, she told me she hated having sex with him. Told me once I had no idea all the terrible things he made her do in bed." A smoldering bitterness weaves its way throughout my body as my stomach and throat constrict. "As if I had no idea what he liked to do in bed…" I take a small sip of water, crush the paper cup, and toss it into the trash. "Mom's the one who told me to lie to the police, not Dad. Mom had all the control, all the power. Without her, the back rubs, the barn, none of it would've happened. I know I shouldn't hate her, but—" I stop abruptly. "I know it's wrong to hate."

"Do you think it's wrong to feel what you feel?" Maureen asks.

I consider her question carefully. "I guess even God hates—I mean—He hates sin." I pause, then choose to venture out in truth. "Honestly? I truly hate her." I wait, and when hellfire doesn't rain down on my head, I continue. "I think I've hated her for a long time."

It is quiet for few moments. My heart is looking all around for God's condemnation, but it cannot find it. I wonder, could He understand me?

"Once," I continue bravely, "when I was ten, I remember Mom talking to a lady from church with a new baby who had colic. Mom said I, too, was a colicky baby, and how I'd never breastfeed. I remember thinking—even at ten years old—that I couldn't stand my mom even as an infant. I can't tell you how many times I wished her dead, but it was a lot."

"So there's a lot of hate there. Any other feelings?" Maureen probes.

"B-b-betrayed," I stammer, looking out the window behind Maureen. "She could've stopped it."

"She betrayed you when you were a defenseless child—a little girl."

"Yes," I murmur, as my tears begin. "Yes, she did."

"And that's hard," Maureen confirms.

Grabbing a tissue, I dry my eyes. "It's hard when I think about it. I mean, I know people say she's my mom, and she loved me and did the best she could, blah, blah, blah. But if that's love, I don't want it. If that's a mom, I don't want one. Maybe that's why I don't think about her, because if I did, I'd just start crying, and I don't know if I could stop. I have to work and try to at least act normal. I can't afford to feel sorry for myself."

"Liz," Maureen speaks delicately now. "What would it be like to feel sad for something lost or something you never had?"

I clear my throat in hopes of getting my question out before I start crying again. "How long would I feel sad?" I take in a deep breath. "If it's forever, I'm not sure I could handle that."

"I don't know how long you'd feel sad, but it wouldn't go on forever, and it wouldn't go on at the same level of intensity. In my work with survivors of sexual abuse," Maureen continues, "one thing they have in common is they don't feel like they can feel sorry for themselves. People are always telling them to 'get off the pity pot,' or 'pick yourself up by your bootstraps.'"

"Or, 'it's all in the past,'" I contribute.

"Yes." She nods. "But the truth is, a big part of healing includes feeling sad for yourself—for what was lost or for what you never had."

I consider her words. "'Sad for yourself' doesn't sound as bad as feeling 'sorry for yourself.' It doesn't sound so *permanent*. If I wouldn't feel sad forever, I could try going back there, emotionally I mean. I just don't want to get permanently lost in despair."

"It's not permanent, but it's a deeply painful realization."

"Maybe I could let the sadness in a little at a time? So it wouldn't overtake me?"

"Absolutely," Maureen assures. "You're in charge of your healing. You're the one in control."

"Being in control is good," I reply. "Different, but good."

SEVEN

Discipline

Irritable and short-tempered most of the day, Mom already longed for school to be back in session. It was the end of June.

Elizabeth, unable to please her, felt the same as she quietly counted out the silverware for the family's evening meal.

"Take out the trash," Mom directed, heaving a sigh as she peeled the potatoes.

Liz carefully hid her annoyance, but inwardly she seethed. Taking out the trash was the boys' job; they were not required to help with dishes or laundry, and they never took turns with Dad. She took care to turn completely away from her mother before rolling her eyes and walking toward the brown paper grocery bag that served as the family's wastebasket.

A sharp pain shot from the nape of her neck as a fistful of her blond hair was grabbed from behind.

Elizabeth froze.

"That's it!" Mom growled through clenched teeth, whipping Elizabeth around by her hair then releasing her violently, shoving her daughter against the kitchen wall. "I've had enough of your disrespect! Get upstairs and write Ephesians six, the whole chapter, five times!"

"W-w-what?"

"W-w-w-what?" her mother mocked. "I ask you to take out the trash, and you sigh like you're goddamned Cinderella! What do you think I do while you're in school sitting on your ass all day? I cook! I clean! I do laundry! Jesus! Do I sigh about every little thing I do?"

Elizabeth stared at her, unblinking.

"So you want to stare," Mom gritted her teeth as she spoke, simultaneously moving closer toward her daughter, arm cocked.

Reflexively jerking her arm upward as her mother struck, Elizabeth deflected a blow intended for her face.

Mom stumbled, then caught herself on the kitchen counter. "You?!" she screeched indignantly. "If I want to slap you, I will slap you! Do you hear? You will obey! Now move your arm!"

Liz lowered her arm, willed it to remain at her side, and waited for the blow.

The force of her mother's fist against her face sent her sprawling headlong into the kitchen table, overturning a chair as she fell to the floor. Tears pooled in the glare she shot back at her mother.

"Go on and stare, Missy," her mother decreed. "We'll see who wins this one. You've just earned yourself a trip to the barn. Now get upstairs."

Still on the floor, Elizabeth eyed the knife drawer just to the right of the silverware drawer. Unmoving, praying her mother would come at her again so she would have reason to kill her, Elizabeth tensed, each tendon, each ligament, each fiber of her body begging for release. An image of hell flashed as the words of Moses came to her: *Thou shalt not kill.*

"Get your ass upstairs and start writing," her mother spat.

Rising stiffly and exiting the kitchen, she grabbed her Bible from the dining room table. Foraging for some lined notebook paper and a pencil from the coffee table, she next made her way to her bedroom and eased onto her bed. Placing the paper on top of her Bible, she began writing. There was no need to look up Ephesians six. She knew it by heart.

Children, obey your parents in the Lord: for this is right. Honour thy father and mother; which is the first commandment, with promise, that it may be well with thee, and thou mayest live long on the earth...

She knew her father would be home any minute, and her stomach knotted. Her head was throbbing from the earlier blow. She placed her Bible beside the pillow away from the edge of the bed and lay her head down. Smothering her face in her pillow, she noticed her mother's cross-stitching on the pillowcase. Raising her head up, she picked up the embroidered section, wiped her nose on it, and threw the pillow to the floor.

She squeezed her eyes shut in chagrin as she heard the gravel churn beneath the wheels of the family station wagon. He was home.

Elizabeth heard the back door open and listened to her mother's report.

"Your fair-haired little angel—I ask her to do one thing, one! And what do I get? Disrespect! The trash! Is that asking a lot? Is it?"

Elizabeth cursed herself for being her father's favorite. In times like these, it made her situation worse. The downstairs conversation gave way to ominous footsteps ascending the staircase to Elizabeth's room.

She sat up on the bed and awaited her sentence.

Her father appeared with her mother behind him. "Lizzie," he began, "what's this about you not obeying your mother?"

"I d-don't know," she began, sniffling. "I thought William was s-supposed to t-take out the trash because I do the d-dishes—"

"Are you the one running this household, young lady?" her mother charged. "Let me answer that question since you don't know. No, you are not. I am. You are here to obey, nothing more."

"I was g-going—" she began. "I mean, I had m-my hands n-near the b-b-bag—"

"What?" her father asked, turning to his wife. "I thought she refused."

Shaking her head no, Elizabeth took a breath. "I w-was, I almost had the p-paper bag, I mean, m-my hands were—"

"Wait a minute," interrupted her mother as an irritated sigh hissed through her teeth. "Here we go again, eh, Elizabeth?

You're going to say you were going to obey me as the Bible commands—immediately and gladly?"

"I-I'm sorry, but I w—" began Elizabeth.

"Oh my," interrupted her mother again. "*Now* you're sorry. Funny, been home all day and haven't heard that one, Del. Oh, but wait! *Daddy's* home and his favorite daughter has decided to apologize in front of him."

Elizabeth dropped her gaze to the floor, and the humming sound came forth like a comforting distant thunder. She honed in on the white windowsill beyond her parents.

"I said, answer me!" her mother yelled, crossing her arms and leaning forward.

Elizabeth looked up.

"That's it! Take her to the barn."

Dad sighed. "Okay, let me change my clothes."

The whole world hesitated.

This was not the routine. He never changed his clothes before the barn because he complained he got all sweaty. He *always* waited until after the barn to change his clothes. He would not be changing his clothes now unless he wasn't going to give her the barn!

Glancing at her father, she wondered if God was trying to reach him. Maybe her mother would fall down the stairs and die. Maybe her mother would burn in hell.

As her parents reached the bottom of the stairs, Elizabeth eased off the bed and headed for the staircase, stopping just before the threshold.

"Becky," Dad began. "Come off it. Who likes to take out the trash gladly? Isn't it enough that she was going to do it? She almost had her hands on the bag for Christ's sake!"

"Don't you dare defy me in front of her," her mother hissed. "She might trick you with her blue eyes and blond hair, but she's not fooling me. She's a conniving—"

"Fine!" he barked. "I've been working since five this morning, and I don't want to hear it, okay? Liz! Get down here!"

Her legs trembled like gelatin as she hurried the rest of the way to the steps where Dad was threading his belt from his blue jean belt loops. He was not going to change his clothes.

Her punishment was imminent.

By the time she reached the back door, her father was already ten steps ahead of her, storming toward the barn.

The whimper escaping her lips must have annoyed him, because he wheeled around, marched back, grabbed her arm, and hurried her to the barn. Shoving her inside, he slid the red planked door closed. She watched as he folded the black belt end to end.

The setting sun cast oblong slants of light through the barn-door planks, illuminating the darkened room in eerie horror. His belt, doubled and held within his great fist, hung black and looming from across the room.

He was angry and tired.

Elizabeth, wide-eyed, stood frozen in her terror. As she locked eyes with her dad, she realized she'd made a serious error. God had chosen to ignore her. Or punish her. Like her parents, God did as He pleased.

He opened his mouth and spoke. "Run."

A simple, routine word. He said it the same way every time. Jogging toward her, right arm midair, black belt twitching, it began.

She had not made it even halfway around when the cracking belt stung her left calf, and she leaped like a deer. Her eyes, squinting in the dimness, found the path as a second crack stung her arm.

She screamed. "Daddy! Da—" Her screams cut short by successive strikes kept ending on guttural notes. She gasped for breath as the next lash struck her back, dead center. His recoil was quick, and the next one struck her left arm. Blood specks emerged upon contact. In heated chase, he swung his belt wildly as she raced around the familiar circle.

Screaming. Running. Screaming. Running.

Her skin tingled, raw and burning from the lashes that striped her back, legs, and arms. The next strike came close to her head, and she wondered if she'd die if the belt buckle hit her hard enough. God commanded His children to obey so they would live long on the earth; if she died as a result of her own disobedience, she would go to hell.

Legs crumbling beneath her, she collapsed in the dirt. Grabbing her knees with her left arm and pulling them to her chest, she shielded her face and head with her right arm, awaiting the next blow.

"Get up." He was panting over her, his palms resting on his thighs.

She made herself as small as possible and tried to speak.

"I c-c-c—" She stopped. She knew God was punishing her for wishing her mother dead. Her parents were righteous people, a husband and wife admired by the church, rooted in God. Everyone said so.

Still panting, her father released the belt, and it fell to the earth.

"You're done," he said breathlessly, extending his hand. "Gimme your hand."

She extended her quivering hand, and he drew her close, encompassing her trembling frame. His hands brushed the wounds on her triceps and she flinched as her breathing continued in short, rapid gasps.

Dropping to his knees, he eyed the top of her shoulders and found them unmarked. Placing his hands atop her shoulders he spoke, this time drawing her head to his shoulder. "Okay now, stop. Take a deep breath."

She obeyed, inhaling as he stroked her long, blond hair. It was her first hug outside of the bedroom in over a week, and she drank in his affection. Moments later, her face nuzzling his neck, she was overcome, and her voice, raw with emotion, interrupted the blackness. "I l-love you D-Dad," she gasped. If only her mother hadn't bullied him so. He hadn't even wanted to give her the barn.

"I love you, too," he replied. "God disciplines His children because He loves them. I'm commanded to do the same. You know that, right?"

Nodding her head, she clung desperately to him, not ready for the affection to end.

"Now," he said, pushing her away then tapping her nose affectionately. "Go. And apologize to your mother."

She waited as he rose to his feet and slid the barn door open. Hurrying past him and into the house, she scaled the steps to her bedroom.

Standing with her back toward the full-view mirror, she raised her shirt, craning her neck for a better view. She counted at least six pink, raised welts on her back, the two in the middle overlapping and revealing fresh blood specks. Two more stripes accentuated her bony ribs, and looking down she saw two more rectangular welts on her right calf—the imprint of her father's belt buckle. A number of smaller stripes marked her calves and behind her knees, in the soft sensitive part.

Her arms were striped with a variety of welts, and dirt had already made its way into the tiny blood-specked crevices. Touching a small, hardened knot alongside her head, she winced at its tenderness. Puzzled for a moment, she didn't remember her father hitting her there. She then remembered falling into the kitchen chair.

Returning to the kitchen moments later, she paused in the entryway.

"I'm s-s-sorry," she said.

"You should be," her mother retorted. "Now finish setting the table."

A ringing telephone accompanied Elizabeth as she approached the utensil drawer. Opening the knife drawer—just enough to capture a glint of steel—she was comforted. She left the knife drawer open, glancing at it periodically, now smiling as she completed the table setting.

"Hello? Oh, hi Doris," said her mother. "No, no one's hurt. You must've overheard the kids' ball game out back. Bob's on his way? I'll send him back in time for his supper. No, no problem at all."

Looking out the kitchen window, Elizabeth saw Bob Jennings crossing the rural highway and heading for her house. Hanging up the phone, her mother approached her husband, now on the couch watching the news. She leaned down to whisper in his ear, and he suddenly stood and went outside.

Elizabeth made her way toward the trash bag. If she took the trash out now, Bob Jennings would see the welts on her arms and legs. He might call the welfare people. She might get to go live with a foster family, like that new girl in her church.

"Where do you think you're going?" her mother asked, reentering the kitchen.

"J-just taking out the t-t-trash?" she stammered.

"Um, no you're not," her mother decreed, enunciating the last consonant. "You're going to your room and putting on some pants and a long-sleeve shirt. It's cooling off."

Under her mother's watchful eye, Elizabeth started for her bedroom. Her mother followed, waiting at the stairwell as Elizabeth donned her jeans and a long-sleeved shirt.

"I haven't got all day," her mother barked, irritated.

Zipping her jeans, she met her mother at the bottom of the stairs. Together they returned to the kitchen. Through the kitchen window, Elizabeth saw Bob Jennings heading back toward his home.

"Elizabeth?" said her mother.

"Yes, ma'am?"

"When Mr. Jennings gets in his driveway, you may take out the trash."

EIGHT

Versions

"How are you doing?" Maureen asks. "Okay?"

I nod.

"Good. Can we backtrack a little? Earlier you said your mom had all the power. Can you tell me more about that?"

"She controlled everything—the back rubs, chores, discipline—all of it. Dad was the head of the household as the Bible commanded, but he wasn't the actual disciplinarian—Mom was. Dad physically gave me the barn, but Mom ordered it up. He never beat me unless Mom made him."

"What's 'the barn'?" she asks.

"It was where we went for discipline. Mom decided who went, and Dad carried out the punishment. We'd go to the barn, he'd slide the door shut, take off his belt, and say, *run*. There was a

39

worn path, an actual 'run,' you could call it. The rules were to stay on the path and run as fast as you could to get the fewest lashes."

"So the rule was to stay on the path as he'd run after you." She pauses, shaking her head. "And he was holding his belt and trying to hit you?"

"Yes. I had to stay on the path. Afterward, he'd hug me and tell me he loved me. The Bible says that God disciplines His children because He loves them, and that's why Dad disciplined me."

"How often did this happen?"

"It depended on Mom's mood. She picked on Em the most. I was next, then Todd. I don't think Will, Sarah, Rachel, or Ruth ever got the barn."

"Why do you think that was?" she asks.

"I think it depended on who Mom hated most. I think she hated Em the most, then me, then Todd."

"And you said earlier that you were your father's favorite?" she asks.

"Yes, and still am."

"And you think this because…"

"He t-told me I was."

"So he told you that you were his favorite," she murmurs. "And he beat Emma the most, then you, and then Todd? And he didn't beat William, Sarah, Rachel, or Ruth?"

I consider her comment as I jot down *he beat you less than Emma, but more than Todd?*

"If he loved me the best, he could've refused to give me the barn." I pause. "I guess I'm not sure the beatings matter when it comes to determining how much Dad loved me, because they were more Mom's doing. D-dad never initiated a beating, only Mom."

"So your mom ordered the beatings, and your dad carried out the order."

"Yes, the beatings were like the back rubs—if not for Mom, neither would have happened."

A quiet confusion is settling upon me. *Why did he beat me more than Todd? Was it because he loved me more? No, that'd mean he loved Emma the most. Why did I have to give the most back rubs? Does that prove he loved me more or Mom hated me most?*

"Based on what you've heard, Maureen"—I clear my throat— "do you think I was Dad's favorite?"

"I don't know, Liz. You may have been, but I think it's worth exploring."

"There are so many possible versions! Sarah told me once that Dad told her *she* was his favorite. I always thought he said that to spare her feelings. Dad *always* told me I was his favorite. He said he doesn't remember anything about the back rubs, because he was in a lot of pain and Mom drugged him up, so he had no idea who was in his bed.

"Now, Dad's sister says the back rubs were mom's fault because she drugged him and never gave him sex.

"And then Todd says it never happened at all, while my grand-mother, my mom's mom, says if I hadn't worn short shorts, it wouldn't have happened in the first place."

I shake my head. "And I was there the whole time, and I still don't know what to believe."

"That must be a difficult way to live."

41

I wonder, is there any other way to live?

"Liz, what do *you* know, so far? Try not to factor in what anyone else thinks. What is your truth?"

"I'm not sure. But I'm holding on to one thing—what you said about it not being my fault—that's all I know for sure right now."

Maureen nods. "I think that is a good place to start."

NINE

Family Night

"I would like to draw your attention to the front please," Mr. Morgan announced, picking up his yardstick and tapping beneath two words written in white chalk.

"Family Night," he began, "is just around the corner." Laying the yardstick upon the chalkboard ledge and folding his arms across his chest, he scanned his fifth grade class in anticipation.

"This year for Family Night, Sunfield Elementary School is honoring our American flag, otherwise known as Old Glory. There will be veterans in the crowd, people who fought for our country, our freedom."

Making his way toward the ordered rows of students, he began weaving between the desks, leaving a comforting scent of Old Spice in his wake.

"We need a representative from our class to read a poem honoring our flag—a volunteer." All eyes followed him. "Whoever reads the poem will be in many ways like our veterans, volunteering with bravery and courage. Do I have any volunteers in my classroom?"

Hands shot up from all over as his words spun like hula hoops in her brain: *bravery and courage.* Oh, how she wanted Mr. Morgan to think she was these things.

So the girl who stuttered did something extraordinary. She raised her hand.

"It's a privilege to represent our class, and this isn't a decision I'll make lightly."

In the profound silence that followed, she nearly jumped out of her seat when his large, gentle hand touched down upon the crown of her head.

"Liz, my girl?" he asked with dignity. "Are you up for the challenge?"

Grinning and cocking her head to the right, she nodded. Awash in the glow of his touch, she realized he had called her "his" girl.

* * *

Three short sentences comprised the Family Night poem. Striving not to stutter, she practiced, practiced, and practiced. She could not recite one sentence fluently, much less three. Overcome with fear as Family Night approached, she decided to confess her failure to Mr. Morgan now rather than disappoint him during the performance.

The next morning she got off the school bus, hurried through the still hallways, and entered his doorway as he graded papers at his desk. He looked up and smiled. "Good morning, my dear." He laid down his pen. "And are we ready for tonight?"

Easing her backpack to the floor, she approached him, speaking to him from across his desk.

"Th-that's why I'm h-here. I keep p-p-practicing, but I k-keep stuttering."

He motioned for her to come around the desk, and as she did, he tenderly took her two small hands and sandwiched them between his two large hands.

"Dear One," he began, "did I ever ask you not to stutter?"

Perplexed, she looked at him.

"You know, Liz" he said, "you don't have to be perfect—no one's perfect except the Good Lord Himself. You just have to do your best. And if you do that, I'll just burst wide open with pride!"

She didn't have to be perfect? She just had to do her best? He would be proud of just her best?

"What do your folks say?" he asked.

"Th-they don't know," she stammered.

"Well, they're in for a treat," he said. "I believe in you. You know that, don't you?"

Comforted by his reassurance, she nodded, smiling.

"So what do you think? Can you do it?" he asked.

She nodded again.

"That's my girl." He smiled.

Pushing up on her toes, she grinned at him. Maybe she *could* do it.

Her day flew by, and soon she was home, brushing her hair in preparation for her big night.

"Do we have to go, Beck?" she overheard her father. "I'm exhausted."

"I have a part!" Elizabeth shouted from the bathroom. "I have to go!"

Five minutes later Elizabeth and her parents were in the car while the younger children stayed at home with Todd in charge.

They arrived at school, one car in a great line of cars, turn signals flashing in dissonance as neon lights reflected off the four-foot-high snowdrifts corralling the freshly plowed parking lot. Exiting the car and hurrying inside the gym, her parents joined the crowd still packing in the folding chairs.

Elizabeth walked to the bleachers as the minutes ticked toward seven o'clock. A brief announcement and then the piano came to life with the opening song, "My Country 'Tis of Thee."

Index card in hand, Liz waited for the last refrain—her cue to descend the bleachers. Her lines were memorized—she didn't need the index card, but holding it provided her with a sense of importance and comfort.

She noticed the children below her parting, making a path for her. Her quivering legs made the short trek down the bleachers then up the gray steps and to the grand stage. Stooping to the floor and picking up the black and silver microphone, she faced the crowd.

She took in a deep breath. "The *r* in r-r-r—" She was forced to stop because she ran out of breath. She took another breath and closing her eyes, tried forcing the word out.

"R-red!" The word exploded into the microphone.

Scanning the crowd for Mr. Morgan, she spied him standing near the stage. He acknowledged her now-frightened eyes with a supportive smile and thumbs-up.

Taking another breath, she tried to relax her throat like she had practiced in speech therapy with Mrs. Wilson.

"—is f-f-f-f-for re-re-respect." She finished the first sentence.

Looking at what now seemed like a mountain of words on the index card, she glanced again toward Mr. Morgan. He winked at her.

Nodding at him, she pursed her lips. She didn't have to be perfect. She had only to do her best.

"The *w* in w-w-w-white," she stuttered and then took another deep breath, "is f-f-f-for w-w-wisdom." Gasping, she saw now there was one line left and took a last, huge breath.

"And the *b* in b-b-blue st-st-st-stands for b-b-bravery." She exhaled victoriously.

The part that should have taken fifteen seconds had taken a full minute, but she was too relieved to be ashamed. She exhaled again and felt her shoulders lighten. Bending down, she laid the microphone upon the wooden stage.

She saw Mr. Morgan jogging up the gray steps toward her, and it was then that she heard the applause.

After hugging her shoulders, he stepped away, extending his right arm toward her as if she were a great performer. Feeling elegant in her blue denim jumper, she curtsied, and the crowd's heartfelt laughter burst forth.

Exiting the stage, she took her place on the bleachers.

Family Night ended, and the initial wave of students exited the bleachers, forming miniature tributaries toward parents, grandparents, aunts, and uncles.

Elizabeth was met simultaneously by Mr. Morgan and her parents. As Mr. Morgan placed his right arm around her shoulders, she grinned. Inhaling his hug, she looked at the floor.

Smiling, Mr. Morgan spoke over the din. "How about our girl?!"

"We didn't know she had such a large part," her mother replied.

"I know!" boomed Mr. Morgan, winking at Elizabeth. "What a surprise for you both!"

She leaned against her teacher, and her right forearm became the conduit through which love flowed openly and without reservation.

"We've got to be going," said her mother. "We've got six other kids at home."

Mom reached for her, and Elizabeth stiffened. Flinching at her mother's hands upon her shoulders, Elizabeth took her coat from her mother then fell in step with the crowd. Soon after, she darted for the water fountain, out of her mother's clutches.

Glancing over her shoulder on her way, she caught Mr. Morgan's eye.

Waving, he clicked the heels of his black shoes together and saluted her. Giggling and flushing with pleasure, she took a drink. Donning her winter coat, she passed beneath the red neon exit sign.

Outside in the darkness, snow outlined the sidewalks and hung like icing upon the massive, barren maple tree.

The abbreviated Luther clan located their car, and as Elizabeth opened the back door of the station wagon and slid onto the vinyl seat, she didn't notice the cold. An intoxicating warmth coursed through her veins. Her parents were quiet, and for that she was grateful. The night replayed itself in her mind, and she was reminded that Mr. Morgan was proud of her. She was *his* girl. He had called her *brave.*

Lying down in the backseat, she tucked her nose and mouth inside her winter coat beneath the zipper and toward her shoulder, where Mr. Morgan had hugged her.

Ah, there it was—the scent of Old Spice.

Comforted, she snuggled down and fell asleep.

TEN

Brothers and Sisters

We move on to my brothers and sisters: Todd, twenty-six years old; me, twenty-four; Emma, twenty-three; Will, twenty-two; Sarah, twenty-one; Rachel, nineteen; and, Ruth, fourteen years old.

"Growing up, we had two distinct sides. Will, Sarah, and I were on one side, and Todd, Emma, and Rachel were on the other. We used to call them the dark side. Ruthie was too young to be on anyone's side. One side always had to get the upper hand to keep their people safe."

"Getting the upper hand—what did that look like?" Maureen asks.

"Punching," hitting, choking, and hair-pulling—most anything was fair game. Whatever we did, we had to do severely, so the other side was afraid enough to leave you and your people alone."

"Sounds like a gang."

"Pretty much. Todd, my oldest brother…we were always at odds. We're still estranged. He thinks I'm a traitor."

"A traitor?"

"Yeah, once when he was home on furlough, he told me I'd ruined our family. He said, 'You don't tell on your own family. You should've brought it before the church and not made it a legal matter. Emma and Sarah, I get—they were little—but you were sixteen, and you knew better.'"

"How do you feel about him?"

"I'd have to say neutral."

"Neutral?"

"Neutral because of how he was when he was younger."

"So does neutral mean you have mixed feelings toward him?"

"Yes." I pause, impressed by her verbal precision. "Mixed feelings. When he was about eight and I was six, I remember sitting on the kitchen floor while Mom was doing dishes. It was summertime, and Todd came in from picking flowers. He gave me a dandelion on his way to the sink. He tapped Mom on her arm, real soft. He took a step back, and while he was looking at the floor and smiling, he held out the rest of the flowers for her. She took them and put them in a drinking glass with some water. Then he jumped up on the countertop and sat there, talking her ear off while she did dishes." My smile faded. "But over time, Mom changed him; she made him mean."

"How so?" Maureen asks.

"There was this one time when he was in eleventh grade and some kids were bullying him. He couldn't fight back—our religion said we had to turn the other cheek. So one morning he just refused to go to school. He told Mom he'd take the barn instead.

"Mom told him he was going to school, but he wouldn't load his backpack, eat breakfast, anything. Mom got so mad she said he was going to school if she had to slap him into going.

"So she calls us kids into the living room. She gets a kitchen chair, sets it in the middle of the floor, and then tells Todd to sit in it."

I take a sip of water. "So she's talking all about obedience, walking around him as he's sitting in this chair, like she's some lawyer. Then she asks, 'Will you go to school?' and when Todd shook his head no, she cracked him so hard across the right cheek, I thought she was going to snap his neck off. He just sat there—stunned maybe at first? I don't know. Anyway, it went on like that, over and over and over. I remember thinking he was like Christ, just taking it and taking it. She asked if he'd go to school; he'd shake his head no; she'd hit him; quote some Bible verse; ask him again, again, and again. There were red handprints all over his face."

"And the rest of the children were all watching this?" Maureen asks, furrowing her brow.

I nod. "After four or five slaps, all of us are crying. Mom keeps it up and says something like, 'See how he makes all of you cry? He thinks only of himself. All he has to do is obey, and will he?' Todd shook his head, and she hit him again.

"At one point, though, she raises her hand to hit him? And he just snaps. He jumped out of that chair like it was on fire, screaming like some wild animal. All of us screamed at the same time, too. It was so scary. He lunged at her, then grabbed her by the throat and slammed her into the wall, screaming. I never heard anything so awful as that kind of scream. His hair was wet with sweat, and mom's eyes were bulging out of her head. Near the end his voice was hoarse, but he told her, 'If you hit me again, as God as my witness, I *will* kill you.'

"Mom's face was all red, and she peed on herself, but Todd kept squeezing her throat tighter and tighter. I was afraid he was going to kill her. Then I was hoping he'd kill her. And, then I was afraid he'd go to jail for killing her. When he did let her go, she thudded to the floor, gasping and coughing. All of us kids rushed to Todd, everybody still crying, some were still screaming. But he didn't hug any of us back. He had this hollow look in his eyes. He was never the same.

"I don't want him in my life because he's unpredictable, unstable almost. But no matter how he treats me, I can't hold much against him because of who he used to be. The interesting thing is, if he knew I'd forgiven him, he'd laugh and say, 'For what?'"

In my pink chair, I raise my hands, palms up, and shrug. "But I can't hate him."

"You've seen a different side of him, a kinder side," Maureen replies.

"Yes, a tender side. And I'm not God or anything, so I won't pretend to know how God will judge Todd. But God knows who Todd used to be, and who his mom was. So when Todd meets his Maker, I'd like to think God could forgive him. And if Todd's still so full of rage that he laughs at God and says he's done nothing wrong? I can't help but wonder if God might still forgive him. Because that's how kind Todd used to be."

ELEVEN

Bills

"Your dad doesn't understand," Mom explained. "This bill will get paid, just not right now. Hide it under my mattress, toward the middle, so it won't fall out. Then meet me at the dining room table."

Elizabeth obeyed. She was accustomed to hiding the bills from her father. Other approved hiding places included the dryer vent, under the hot-water heater, and behind the washing machine.

Mom gave her a blank piece of paper when she returned to the dining room. "You know how to write in cursive, right?"

Elizabeth nodded.

"Show me. Write 'paid in full' on here."

Elizabeth again complied and made a small heart instead of dotting her *i*.

"Good," Mom praised. "Here, do the same thing on this bill, but without the heart. Just make a normal dot for the *i*."

Elizabeth penned *Paid in Full,* across the electric bill.

Her mother examined the bill. "You have beautiful handwriting," she emphasized. "Now, if your dad asks, there was no mail today except this, okay?"

"Mom?" Elizabeth asked. "I won't g-go to hell for lying to Dad about the b-b-bills, right?"

Mom, still examining the altered bill, shook her head. "Of course not," she replied. "Your job is to obey, nothing more. Besides, if it was a sin, it would fall on my head, not yours."

"Aren't you afraid of hell?"

Mom chuckled. "The Lord knows I'm just taking care of my family. I have no reason to be afraid of hell," she replied. "You'll understand when you're older. Now, don't mention this to your father. We don't want him worrying about the bills, hmm?"

Elizabeth nodded. Worry meant stress. Stress meant migraines. Migraines meant back rubs. "For sure," she affirmed. "The secret's safe with me."

TWELVE

Awareness

Fall 1989, twenty-four years old

"So, today's the day I get to meet your shrink." Matt whispers in my ear, making his eyes wide as we enter the lobby of Maureen's office.

Gasping at his audacity, I punch his left shoulder, and he chuckles.

His joking is a sign he is nervous. At the window, I write out my check for seventy-five dollars. The lady on the other side of the window turns it over and stamps it.

We take a seat in the waiting area. I wonder how many new marriages survive one spouse meeting the other spouse's counselor.

Moments later, Maureen opens the lobby door near the reception desk. I stand, and Matt follows suit.

As we enter her office, I notice the extra chair Maureen has added to our meeting area. He walks toward the pink chair, and I interject.

"Um, that's my chair."

Matt hesitates and Maureen chuckles, extending her hand to the extra wooden chair she has placed adjacent to her chair and mine. "Nice to meet you," she says, extending her hand to Matt. "I'm Maureen."

"Nice to meet you," Matt reciprocates. I place my hands in my lap and look down in the quietness.

"I want to thank you for coming," Maureen begins. "I've heard a lot about you already."

Matt raises his eyebrows, and our eyes lock.

"Mostly good," I offer with a smile, and I wait for him to make a joke. He does not, and I sense he is more comfortable.

Maureen says something about me being hurt as a child. She pauses, and when no one else speaks, continues. "Liz has a great deal of courage. Healing is hard, hard work."

"It's helping," Matt says. His voice sounds strange in a room accustomed to women's tones. "I mean, I don't know what you do or say, or whatever, but it's helping."

Maureen nods. "It's going to take some time."

Nodding, he looks my way, smiling one of his "it's okay" smiles.

"I think she's talking years," I interject.

Matt pauses. "Whatever it takes," he replies. "You know that, Liz, right? Whatever it takes?"

I nod, wondering if he already knew it would take years.

"Do you have any questions, Matt?" Maureen asks.

Shaking his head no, he stands.

Maureen also stands. She shakes his hand again. "Again, thanks for coming, Matt."

I smile at him. "Yes, Matt. Thanks for coming to see my shrink."

He turns and smiles at me, then glances toward Maureen as if to gauge her reaction.

Maureen is smiling and her eyebrows are raised.

He closes the door behind him.

I heave a sigh of relief. "That was relatively painless."

Maureen's gentle smile pops up. "You expected otherwise?"

"I didn't know what to expect," I chuckled, opening my notebook.

"So you're okay with how it went?"

"Yes, relieved actually."

"Good. I see you already have your notebook open."

"Yes, two things if we have time."

"We have plenty of time, Liz. Go ahead."

"I noticed something with Dad this weekend," I begin. "He came over to help us move from the apartment to our new place. As we're loading some boxes into our new car, he says, 'I'll drive your new car to the new place, Lizzie. We'll ride together.' Then, a few minutes later I hear him in the kitchen talking to Matt. He says, 'Matt, do you mind if Liz and I take the new car? We'd like to ride together.' He asked Matt's permission, but not mine. And I never said I wanted to ride with him. He just made up what I said I wanted."

"So your dad asked for Matt's permission to use the new car, but he made the decision for you."

"Yes, and it happens all the time. I just don't think I've ever noticed it."

"Do you know why you're noticing it now?"

I lean my head back against the pink chair for a moment. "I think it's because I'm not so afraid of him…well, not just of him. I'm not so afraid all the time in general. I think I'm less afraid now than I've ever been—as a child or an adult."

"So you're feeling less afraid. Would you say your mind is freed up when it's not so afraid? Does that fit?"

"Yes," I reply, nodding as I take a moment to write in my journal. *I'm less afraid these days.*

"Okay, number two. This one might sound strange, but I feel like it represents my life to a T. I went through a fast-food drive-through and extended my hand to give the guy my money. The guy leans out the window, extends his hand, but passes over the money in my hands and instead caresses my upper arm, then my elbow, then my wrist. The guy's whole head is hanging out the drive-through window and he's stretching his neck out, looking at my legs. As his hand goes back toward my palm, he takes the money and says, 'Nice legs.' And I just sat there."

"What were you feeling?" Maureen asks.

"Afraid."

"And what were you thinking when he was touching your arm?"

"I don't think I was thinking. I tried to be still and quiet. There's nothing I could do anyway, so I just waited until it was over."

"There's nothing you can do anyway." Maureen mirrors. "So you waited until it was over."

I nod.

"Like when you were a child," she says.

"Yes," I say, "but I'm an adult now—a married adult. I feel unfaithful to my marriage when I act this way."

"I think you froze in fear," she replies.

Her words fit like the perfect pair of winter gloves.

"You said you were feeling afraid," she continues. "What did you want while you were feeling afraid?"

"For him to stop. I just wanted it to be over."

"What did you do when he said you had nice legs?"

"I looked down at my legs and wondered if my shorts were too short."

"So you wondered if you'd done something wrong."

I nod.

"Liz, it's not your fault. And it sounds like the signals you send when you get an unwanted advance aren't what you'd like."

"Yes, I send out the wrong signals," I concur.

"So you want to send out different signals? Signals that say 'stop what you're doing'?" Maureen asks.

I nod, imagining I can be that powerful.

"What if you had a plan?" she suggests. "You wouldn't have to use it, but it could be on the shelf, to use if you wanted."

"A plan sounds good," I agree.

"Any ideas?" she asks.

Pausing in the silence, I shake my head. "None."

"You have some options, and none of them is wrong," she encourages.

I pause for a moment. "I could say no?"

"That's a good start," she replies.

"What if I stutter?"

"No means no, whether or not you stutter. The meaning is the same," she shrugs.

"True. And it's one word," I chime. "Maybe I won't stutter."

Maureen leans forward just a little. "And maybe you won't think about stuttering or not stuttering. Maybe you'll be a little angry that someone violated your personal space."

I chuckle, shaking my head. I bet Maureen didn't take violations on her personal space sitting down.

"At least I'll be doing something besides freezing," I conclude, finishing up my notes. "There," I announce, looking up. "My list is done."

"Okay," Maureen replies, glancing at the clock. "We have a few minutes left. I have something I'd like you to try if you're up to it. A kind of homework assignment."

I nod at her, curious.

"You've shared that it's hard to remember chunks in your childhood; how it's like a slide show?"

"Yes. Some things I remember vividly, others partially, but then some slides are a white, blank slate."

"Sometimes," Maureen reveals, "the mind takes over in an act of self-protection. We're all wired to survive, and the brain has a unique way of doing its part to make sure we do that. Some experts think the mind allows us to remember things when we are ready, when we can safely remember them. So I'd like you to think about what it'd be like to be a child raised in a family like yours—a little girl with no way out, no options except to obey her parents, trapped in a place she calls home."

"I can try that. How do I—" my voice trails off.

"Get started?" she asks.

I realize she's done this before.

"You could start by making sure you have some uninterrupted time. Sit someplace comfortable. Then think about this little girl in your family. Close your eyes and try to go there with her. No rules," she finishes.

"Sounds easy enough," I say.

"It might be easy, Liz, and it might not. We can always evaluate afterward."

I close my notebook then rise to leave. "I like having that idea on the shelf. Thanks."

"You're welcome," Maureen replies.

Exiting, I wonder if there will ever be a time I leave her office feeling less afraid than when I came in.

THIRTEEN

Reciprocity

Sighing, Elizabeth poured milk over her wheat puffs. She hated wheat puffs; she hated cutting wood on Saturdays; and she hated that everyone in the family helped cut wood except her mother.

"I don't mind doing the dishes, girls, since you'll be cutting wood all day," her mother announced.

Emma rolled her eyes as a respectful "thank you," dripped from her lips.

Masking her own resentment, Elizabeth placed her cereal bowl in the sudsy kitchen water. *Ten minutes of doing dishes inside a warm house versus eight hours cutting wood in the cold,* she begrudged on her way to the coat room.

Elizabeth donned her snow pants alongside Emma, William, Sarah, and Rachel. The roar from the truck's engine and a whirl of snowflakes burst through the back door as their father entered.

"Becky?" he yelled.

His wife poked her head out of the bathroom door, hairbrush in hand.

"You'll have to drive the girls up in the station wagon. They can't ride in the truck bed today—wind chill's too cold. The boys and I'll be leaving now. Give us about five minutes to make a path with the truck to the woodshed."

"That'll be fine," called their mother.

The back door opened again, and a snow-covered Todd appeared.

"All set, Dad," he said. "I put gas and oil in both saws."

"Good," his father answered, tossing the sixteen-year-old the car keys. "Warm up the wagon for your mom. And Becky, you're bringing lunch at twelve?"

"Twelve it is," she replied.

By 8:15, Ruth was wrapped in a wool blanket and given to Elizabeth, now sitting glumly in the backseat. The woodshed was a mile away and by 8:25, their mother was following the path made by the Chevy truck, avoiding the three-feet-high snowdrifts on each side of the wheel wells. Just outside the woodshed she shifted the car into park, looking over her right shoulder toward Elizabeth.

"Put Ruthie up here so Rachel can hold her—Rachel's staying home today. It's too cold. She's been sick once already this week, and the last thing we need's another doctor bill. Tell your dad she's with me, would you, Liz?"

"Sure," Elizabeth murmured, opening her door as Rachel also opened hers. Elizabeth plopped Ruth in the front seat upon Rachel's lap.

Slamming the door closed, she stood watching as her mother backed out the station wagon, turned, and headed for home.

Joining ranks behind Emma and Sarah, five silent figures followed their father, single file, about two hundred yards along the snow-covered path to a clearing. The blustering wind accompanied their squeaking boots upon the blinding white snow.

"Okay!" Their father shouted over the wind, surveying his work crew, "William and girls, move this brush to the big pile. Todd, I'll have wood for you to split in a minute." He paused for a moment, raising his scarf over his mouth and nose as he looked up at the frosty skyline. "I wish the sun would come out," he said, his voice muffled. "Todd, get the truck and bring it up here so if anyone's cold they can get out of the wind. Hey!" he shouted, startling the children. "Where's Rachel?"

"Oh, Mom said it's t-too cold for her since she's been sick," Elizabeth replied.

"Your mother's right about that," Dad agreed. "Okay, let's get moving." He grabbed the chainsaw and pulled the rope cord.

Roaring to life, the chainsaw startled a small flock of crows. They burst into the sky like black fireworks.

In quick motions their father began clearing the scrub trees. In an attempt to keep warm, the children pushed themselves to keep moving, hauling the small limbs and brush to the burn pile. By ten o'clock, however, the four younger children were inside the truck cab, out of the winter wind, sitting on each other's laps to stay warm.

The chainsaw stopped, and the children looked to see their father approaching the driver's side window. William rolled the window down, and their father's face, reddened from the cold, accentuated the frozen particles hanging from his nostrils.

"Warmin' up?" he shouted, forgetting the chain saw was off, and he needn't yell.

Heads nodded.

"We need to get this wood loaded," he continued, less loud. "Then we'll head for the shed and cut it—too cold out here in the open. Surprised you kids lasted as long as you did." Wiping his nose on his sleeve he turned toward the woodpile. "Come on, I'll help load," he directed.

"Come on, let's get this over with," Emma moaned, and the children tumbled out of the cab.

Twenty minutes later, the truck bed laden with wood, their father checked his watch.

"Your mother'll be here by noon," he said, brushing a mix of snow and sawdust off his thighs. Raising his right eyebrow, he continued. "If we have this wood cut and stacked by then, I say we'll call it a day and eat lunch at home."

"Yes!" William shouted.

Elizabeth smiled. Suddenly her toes did not seem quite so cold.

Backing the truck into the woodshed, their father killed the engine, and by the time he was out of the cab, the children were lined up and awaiting instructions.

Elizabeth and William were assigned to unload the truck bed. Emma would hold the limbs for her father to cut with the chainsaw into fireplace-sized pieces. Todd, standing with ax in hand, would split the stumps with help from Sarah, who'd steady the wobbly stumps and hand him the wedge when necessary.

The assembly line, soon operating at full throttle, filled the air with sawdust and wood chips. Within forty minutes, the truck bed was emptied.

Their work complete, they sat in the truck bed passing the thermos, quenching their thirst, and washing down sawdust.

"We're eating lunch at the house?" Elizabeth confirmed.

"Right," he confirmed. "We'll let your mom know when she gets here before she starts unloading the car."

"Wanna play Monopoly when we get home?" asked William.

"Yeah!" they all shouted in unison.

A dull rumble emanated from outside the shed, and the kids leaped off the truck bed.

"She's early!" squealed Sarah. "Let's go!"

Running toward the already parked car, Elizabeth paused at the driver's side window as her mother rolled it down.

"Take this," she began, extending a thermos through the window.

"Wait!" said Elizabeth. "Dad says it's too cold to eat up here."

"Too cold in the shed?" her mother asked.

"It's freezing!" said Elizabeth, jumping up and down in glee.

"Beck," said Delbert, now tapping on the passenger's side window. "Too cold today—me and the boys will meet you girls at the house for lunch."

"I gathered that," Mom replied.

Jostling their way inside the warm station wagon, a happy silence descended upon the girls.

"C-can we turn the radio on, please?" asked Elizabeth.

"Sure," said her mother, reaching for the knob.

"We're playing Monopoly after lunch, okay, Mom?" asked Sarah.

"After you do the dishes, sure," responded their mother.

"We thought you were doing dishes," said Elizabeth in genuine surprise.

Their mother paused, clearing her throat. "What I said was, if you worked in the woods *all day* I'd do them. I have other things to do besides dishes."

Elizabeth's mumbled, "Like what?" might have gone unnoticed had the radio's volume been turned up.

"Excuse me?" her mother stated.

"I just said, like what?" said Elizabeth trying to mask her irritation.

"Like what? Like laundry and cooking, that's what," she replied.

Elizabeth rolled her eyes. She and Emma had folded the laundry last night, and lunch was already prepared.

"Satisfied?" her mother asked.

"W-w-what'd you do this morning?' she asked, anything but satisfied.

Sarah and Emma looked away from their eldest sister.

"Excuse me?" her mother replied, her voice an octave higher as she turned off the radio.

"I'm just asking. We worked four hours. What'd you do the past four hours?"

"Young lady, who do you think did all the work while you were in diapers? You think you're too good to help just because you cut a little wood this morning?"

Incensed, Elizabeth bit her tongue. She didn't ask to be born. Maybe if her mother would stop having sex with her father, she'd stop popping out so many kids, and the diaper issue would be done with. Besides, it was not a *little* wood.

"I hid the mail yesterday," Elizabeth trumped, "and told Dad there was none."

Her mother's eyes widened, although she said nothing. Fixing her stare on the snowy roadway, she pulled into their driveway.

"Elizabeth, I'd like to see you in my room," her mother announced as the four doors opened.

"Fine," she replied.

After peeling off her winter layers, Elizabeth hung them on the clothesline in the laundry room and hurried upstairs.

"You know I hide the bills for your father's own good," whispered her mother.

"We cut wood and froze our butts off," argued Elizabeth.

"Watch your mouth," her mother cautioned.

"You're the one who always says, 'one hand w-w-washes the other,'" Elizabeth hissed. "Can't you just help with dishes?"

The two heard their father and the boys enter the house as the wind slammed the door closed behind them.

"Whew! Haven't started eating yet?" their father blustered.

"Not yet," replied Emma.

"I'm going to the bathroom," he said. "Then I'm eating. I'm starved!"

"I'm not asking you to do all the dishes, Mom. Just help—"

"Fine," her mother quipped. "Fine, I see what game you're playing."

"It's not a game, Mom. We're tired and cold and—"

Her mother turned away and headed down the stairs. Elizabeth followed behind her. After lunch, their mother helped clear the table and do dishes and soon, the children were playing Monopoly.

As Elizabeth placed her dog on *Go*, she heard the fourth step creak. Looking up the staircase, she saw her father halfway up the stairway to his bedroom. Thank goodness it wasn't her turn to go first.

Their mother entered the dining room, hands on her hips. "Your father has a migraine, so keep it down. Elizabeth, you're first."

"Not my turn," she answered, "I went last—"

"I know, I know. You went last the last time. But since Emma went first on Wednesday, you're going first today. Meet me in the kitchen for his pills."

In protest Elizabeth tossed her silver dog into the empty Monopoly box lid and entered the kitchen as her mother opened a vial of medicine.

"M-mom—" Elizabeth began.

"I've been thinking," her mother interrupted. "Why don't you tell your father about the bills?" She extracted two white pills from the amber vial. "Let's see if *that* makes his headache go away."

Reaching for another bottle, she opened the top and tapped out a yellow pill. "And don't worry, while you're with your father, I'll try to find some work to do—if I have any to do, that is. Your hand," she directed, dropping the pills onto Elizabeth's outstretched palm.

Elizabeth knew the bills worried her father. Stress meant migraines. Migraines meant back rubs. Eyes downcast, she exited the kitchen. Ascending the stairs like a wraith, she was entranced the moment her foot brushed the first step.

Hearing her name called two hours later, she emerged from his bedroom and walked down the stairwell holding the sides. She stumbled on the last step and fell to her knees. Rising, she walked toward the bathroom, keeping her hands far from her face, ignoring Mom's "How's his headache?"

Her mother, annoyed, hurried upstairs to check on her husband.

Washing her hands with hot soapy water, Elizabeth grappled with the roulette rotation. There were no more guarantees, no more scheduled reprieves, no way of knowing when she'd be next.

Looking in the mirror, she saw herself through a thin, white veil. Like dry ice, her appendages ebbed and flowed without boundaries. Her sheer hand opened the medicine cabinet, twisting off the cap of the rubbing alcohol. A generous amount poured into her right hand, and rubbing her hands together, she coated her arms, neck, and face. She picked up the bottle and emptied the contents upon the front of her shirt. The medicinal scent saturated the air, and she inhaled. The now-empty bottle fell to the floor, rolling hollowly to rest against the wall.

The humming noise called to her from the corner wall of the bathroom, and she walked toward it. Curling up on the floor and facing the white wall, she closed her eyes. As the humming became louder, she entered the wall. Rubbing her fingers together, she welcomed the cool latex paint cascading over her body.

Her mother barged in.

"Next time I ask you—" she began.

Twitching at the smell of her mother's perfume, Elizabeth reached down, grabbed her neckline, and pressed the still saturated collar against her nose with a catatonic force. She inhaled deeply as her still-closed eyes gripped the whiteness. The hollow din of her mother's voice pecked at the cool latex surface of her forehead, then diminished into silence. Still huddled on the floor, she faded away, cloaked beneath the ridges of white latex.

There was a slight pressure beneath her armpits, and then a softness beneath her. From far away a mattress squeaked, a doorknob turned, and a door closed. Still bathing in the warm, luminous glow insulating her from the outside world, she breathed a sigh of comfort.

Perhaps there were some guarantees in life, after all.

FOURTEEN

Perceptions

Fidgeting in my pink chair, I wonder what it must be like to sit listening to people drone on for hours. I can't believe I've never seen Maureen yawn. Opening my notebook, I glance at the number I've written down: sixteen.

"I w-want to tell you something. I w-was little, around nine or ten, I think, when the back rubs started. B-but I was older when the last back rub happened—old enough to maybe have stopped it."

I pause, awaiting her reply.

"So you're saying you think you could have stopped it?"

"I could've at least asked him to stop, or fought him off. But I didn't do anything."

"Okay," she says. "You didn't ask him to stop. And you didn't fight him off. What might have happened if you'd asked him to stop or fought him off?"

"He might have stopped if I'd have just asked him. But I never did my part by asking him."

"So, 'your part,' as you say, means you could have asked him to stop, and he might have stopped sexually abusing you."

"I'll never know if he would've stopped, because I never asked him."

"Do you know if your sisters asked him to stop or fought him off?"

"Sarah told Dad it was wrong, and he said he'd stop. And Emma hit him to make him stop."

"And did he stop?"

"He stopped with Sarah, but not with Emma. But that was *them*. I was his favorite. Wait, wait, I have to stop saying that so automatically. I guess if he stopped with Sarah, then maybe *she* was his favorite?"

Maureen's expression is thoughtful, but she does not reply.

"In foster care, when all of us were together for a visit, both Em and Sarah said Dad told them that *they* were his favorites."

"Do you remember how you felt back then?" Maureen asks.

"I felt sorry for them. I knew Dad said that to make them feel better. I knew he loved me the best. I knew it in my heart. I knew it like I knew the sky was blue."

"So back then, during that conversation with your sisters, you couldn't hear that one of them, or both of them, might have been his favorite. Your reality couldn't accept it?"

"I guess not, because inside I knew they were wrong."

"And now?" she asks.

"I d-don't know. All three of us couldn't have been his favorite. And since he stopped when Sarah asked him, maybe she was his favorite."

"Maybe. Could there be another explanation?"

"Maybe none of us were his favorite? Maybe he said that to keep all of us quiet?" I wonder which is worse—that he didn't love any of us or that he loved one of my sisters more than me?

"You know, I was s-s-s-sixteen the last time we were in bed together."

"And that troubles you?"

I nod once and wonder what she could possibly say to make me feel better about this one.

"Liz, six or sixteen doesn't matter. He was the parent, the adult. You were the child. It wasn't your fault."

Her words allow me to inch forward to a safer place, and I try saying her words aloud to see if they fit.

"So even though I was sixteen and I never asked him to stop and I never tried to fight him off, it's still not my fault? Don't I look cowardly?"

"Liz, you look like you were surviving. You were silent because it was all you were allowed to be. And the fact that you were sixteen means you were able to survive for a long time under horrible circumstances. The child is never responsible for the abuse."

"So"—I add, extending this application—"if it wasn't my fault, I'm not the one who wrecked my family?"

"If you were the one who wrecked your family, you must have been one powerful little kid," Maureen says, widening her eyes. "Your father was the adult, he had the power. You, the child, had no power. And let me share with you, you're not alone in what you're feeling. Many children feel responsible when their family falls apart, even though they have no power to influence the family's ability to stay intact."

"So sixteen doesn't matter to you?" I ask, realizing I sound like a broken record.

"It just doesn't matter," she replies. "Not to me or anyone else who values children."

* * *

Sitting in my driveway, I watch the rain madly pelt the windshield. Craning my neck toward the gray sky, I wonder how long I'll have to wait for the downpour to end.

Opening my journal, I scan my notes: *He was the adult. You were the child. Children are never responsible for the abuse. Six or sixteen, it was not your fault.*

An age-old pattern in my thinking has been interrupted. It's as if my mind has been retooled.

I don't think I'm the one who ruined my family.

Closing my journal, I peer again at the hovering, dark, gray clouds and realize I could be waiting in my car for a long while.

Tucking my journal under my coat, I open my car door and take a step out into the downpour. Pausing, I turn my face upward, and I'm surprised at how warm the rain is. Closing my eyes as it cascades over me, I chuckle aloud at my thoughts.

Go on and rain, then. Let it rain all day, all night, all week. Let some old man say he's going to build an ark, I don't mind. It doesn't matter any to me. I was sixteen and that didn't matter to Maureen. And if it doesn't matter to her, maybe it doesn't matter to God.

And maybe one day, it won't matter to me.

FIFTEEN

Canada

Every summer the family took a week-long vacation to a new camping and fishing spot. This year their destination was a public reserve in Canada.

Twelve hours of driving, and finally they saw the sun's first nod toward the still blue horizon. Towering pine, oak, and birch trees canopied the belabored station wagon as seven children, now on high alert, took turns craning their necks out the two rear car windows, gaping at the Canadian wilderness that would be their home for the next week. Slowing to a stop on the crest of a hill overlooking an enormous lake already shrouded in near dusk, they spied the lone amenity—a weathered picnic table.

Piling out of the car, the boys and their father set to erecting the tent, digging a hole for bathroom purposes, and preparing the boat for fishing.

The girls hung the clothesline and gathered firewood and kindling. Elizabeth and her mother set up the tripod for cooking meals. Within forty-five minutes, the camp was a picture of order and efficiency.

Elizabeth tried to remain pleasant as her father and brothers prepared to take the boat out. She resented that William got to fish with her father first. He was two whole years younger than she was. But her father favored the boys when it came to fishing, and any protest would hinder her goal to fish in the morning.

"Need some night crawlers in case the daredevils don't work?" she offered as they gathered their tackle boxes.

"Hey, yeah!" said her father. "Grab us a dozen or so."

"Make 'em big ones!" shouted William.

Grabbing a flashlight Elizabeth rummaged through the tackle cooler, then removed the small plastic lid with holes in the top. She quickly scooped up the squiggling crawlers placing them into a large Styrofoam cup that already had a hole in the lid. She passed it to Todd, now standing beside the boat. He placed the crawlers in one of the tackle boxes, then pushed off with his bare right foot, taking a great stride back into the boat as it slid away, now gliding upon the rippling water.

Her father pulled the rope cord three times, and the Evinrude motor burbled to life. He glanced at his watch. "It's six now, we'll be home at eight, latest," Del barked.

Waving, Elizabeth turned from the boat and toward her mother, standing near the tripod. The frozen chili she'd packed earlier was just beginning to bubble in the cast-iron camping kettle. Elizabeth offered to get the crackers and bowls.

"Why, aren't you helpful?!" Mom said. "Want to split a soda? You get the soda, and I'll get the cups."

Elizabeth made her way to the cooler and carried the chilled soda bottle back to the picnic table. Her mother had already set out two Styrofoam cups. Elizabeth poured, watching the bubbling fizz fill the top third of the cup with foam. Mother and daughter stood for a moment, each holding their own cup, as tiny waves lapped the sandy shore in a soothing rhythm, and the slight breeze mussed their hair.

The chili simmered for nearly two hours before the faint putter of the boat motor, mingling with excited voices, drew near in almost total blackness.

Running to the crescent-shaped water's edge, the girls stepped aside as the boat slid to a stop in the muddy sand.

"Becky!" Dad yelled. "Look at these fish!"

Taking a lanky step off the side of the boat, Delbert held up the loaded silver stringer where the early moonlight and shadow of the blazing campfire reflected the sparkling scales of four gigantic pike thrashing about, dangling just above the water. Two of the pike were at least forty inches in length. Gasps filled the small inlet as everyone awed at the massive fish.

"Who's going to clean them?" asked their mother, grinning. "That's a lot of fish!"

"Boys?" their father asked.

"No problem," said Todd. "I'll clean them right now if we can fix 'em for dinner tonight."

Mom hesitated. "It's already late, almost eight o'clock. That means it will be an hour before they're cleaned and cooked. And the chili's ready now."

"Tell ya what, Todd. Let's have 'em for dessert," said their father. "I'm too hungry to wait an hour to eat supper."

"Me, too," Todd acknowledged.

"If you can clean them in the next ten minutes, they can cook in some foil while we eat up the chili," affirmed Mom.

Elizabeth sighed amid her parents' peaceful, reasonable nature. Gazing first into the black forest, then up toward first stars embedded within the evening sky. She wondered what kind of magic lived here. Perhaps it might follow them all home.

"Becky," murmured their father, "Get a load of Lizzie."

Both parents chuckled.

"You should've seen her helping out earlier," Mom added. "You'd think she deserved to go fishing in the morning."

"I think that can be arranged," replied Dad.

"Dad!" whined William on his way to the fish pyre. "No fair! It's always better to fish in the morning!"

"If you don't watch your attitude, you'll never know what it's like to fish in Canada in the morning," responded Dad.

Elizabeth toned down her smile. Will was one of her allies.

After the fish were cleaned, Dad filleted them and placed them upon a piece of aluminum foil, topping each fillet with a pat of butter and a sprinkling of salt and pepper. Next, he creased the foil over the top and placed the sealed packets on the iron grate of the tripod. Finally, he lowered the grate so it hung just above the coals.

"Dessert in the making," he pronounced.

Surrounding the glowing fire and tripod, each sitting on their respective stone or stump of wood, the family paused as Dad gave thanks for their safe travel and made a special request for good weather. A chorus of amens followed. Mom dished out the chili and crackers.

"Fishing makes you hungry," said Will at one point, and everyone nodded in agreement.

At nine o'clock, dessert was served. The flaky, tender fish melted in Elizabeth's mouth. William licked the aluminum foil clean.

"Man! This is good, but my hands stink," William announced, placing his fingers beneath Elizabeth's nose. "Take a whiff."

Elizabeth sniffed and then grimaced. Lowering her voice, she put her hands on her hips. "Dead fish aroma," she announced in a masculine tone. "You good hunter!"

The family laughed.

Heavy sighs evidenced great satisfaction, and for a moment the crackling of burning wood was the only sound save the mysterious call of the Canadian loons.

"'Bout bedtime?" asked their father, looking at his wife.

"I'd say so," yawned Mom, stretching her arms overhead. "Come on girls—let's get comfy in the car. The boys are sleeping in the tent. Ruthie's already sleeping in the front seat, so try to be quiet."

"Lizzie, still want to go fishing in the morning?" her father asked, rising.

"Y-yes," she answered.

"Good," he said. "Then you can sleep in the tent with me. That way we can head out without waking anyone up."

"Delbert, we don't have enough sleeping bags," Mom began. "We have three. Tap on the window in the morning. I'm sure she'll be a light sleeper."

"No, we'll wake up the whole camp," Dad insisted. "We can share a sleeping bag, right, Lizzie?"

Elizabeth froze as the humming in her head began. Struggling to answer to avoid appearing thankless, she blinked, nodding her head once.

"There you have it," Dad decreed. "Let's get to bed. Five in the morning comes early."

Rising, the children gathered up their long underwear and an extra pair of socks. Elizabeth sat on an old stump a few feet from the fire, staring at the socks in her hands and the shoes on her feet.

"Liz, get going," Mom said. "You heard your dad. Five o'clock comes early."

"She's just tired, Becky," her father soothed, approaching Elizabeth and rubbing her back. "It's been a long day."

Elizabeth unlaced her shoes, donned her second pair of socks, and after slipping her shoes back on, headed for the tent.

Entering the first of the two rooms, she zipped up the mosquito netting behind her. Eyeing the loaded shotgun propped in the corner, she reminded herself she was safe from the bears. She overheard Todd and William arranging the back room to their liking.

Casing the large room, she saw the black sleeping bag on the tent floor.

Behind her she heard the zipper and turned to see her father poking his head through the doorway.

"Jump on in and warm up the sleeping bag. I've gotta pee." His head vanished.

She slipped off her shoes then climbed inside the sleeping bag. Laying her head down upon the pillow, she watched the dancing shadow flames from the fire rise and fall upon the tent's green canvas fabric.

Her father entered the tent, holding the Coleman lantern. Snuffing out the wick, he set it down near the gun.

"I never knew a girl who liked to fish as much as you," he said, slipping off his shoes. Crouching, he unzipped his side of the sleeping bag.

"Scoot over," he said. "I'm bigger than you, ya know."

Sliding over and onto her side as far as she could to give him room, her mind began to hum louder. Facing the green canvas and away from her father, she supported her head with the elbow of her right arm. Her left arm, a futile barrier, lay across her left hip.

She felt his hairy arm slip beneath her left arm, encircle her waist, and draw her lower back and buttocks to his groin area. Her body quivered.

"Cold?" he whispered, his breath moist and warm in her ear.

"N-no," she replied, swallowing hard.

Resisting the green canvas, her mind faltered. As her father adjusted his pillow, she knew she must hurry. Taking in a deep breath, she stubbornly eased into the green canvas where, to her surprise, the humming noise didn't seem to mind the green at all.

Rubbing her middle finger and thumb together, she felt the rough, cool canvas between her fingers.

Relieved, she blinked, and the humming noise began its ascent, silencing her father's breathing in her ear. Her back, now to the campfire, was warmed by the fire's flames. As the elastic on her flowered bra lifted upward away from her skin, she focused on the back of her eyelids, and the humming rose to a deafening level.

And in the cool night of the Canadian air, Elizabeth remembered nothing more.

* * *

The first rays of sunshine danced upon her cheek and the tent floor near her head. A loon called out, and she awakened, smelling ash from last night's now-smoldering fire.

"We overslept," said her father, disappointed. "Let's get fishing, Lizzie."

SIXTEEN

Lies

I clear my throat and hold up one finger.

Will my revelation forever change my relationship with Maureen?

"One today?" she asks.

"I lie," I say, cutting to the chase.

"Okay. You lie. Can you give me an example?"

"Um, plenty. As a kid I lied and said it wasn't my turn when it was. Last week I lied to Dad about how much I'm working. Yesterday I lied to Matt about how much I spent grocery shopping." I pause. "The worst thing about lying is you lose trust. When you lie to someone, they won't know if they can trust you again. And lying is a major sin; God hates a liar and has a special place in hell just for liars. Satan himself is the father of lies." I stop here, breathless.

"You worry you'll lose trust."

"Do you still trust me, knowing I lie?"

"Good relationships require trust, and I can see you care about trust."

I don't think I'll ever lie to Maureen. I pay her too much money. Should I tell her this?

"I do trust what you tell me, Liz. And what you're telling me," she adds, "is that you lie, and it bothers you."

"Thank you," I say, grateful that she has named it.

"You're welcome." She smiles. "Let's slow down and take a look here, one at a time. The first one you mentioned was lying about saying it wasn't your turn?"

I nod.

"It's sometimes helpful to look at what you're feeling when you tell a lie. Do you remember what you were feeling when you said it wasn't your turn?"

"I don't know if there is a feeling word. I just wanted out of the back rubs, the sexual abuse."

"Do you think there's anything wrong with wanting out of sexual abuse?"

"No," I answer with certainty. "No, but lying is a major sin. I don't know why I chose to lie."

"If lying was the *only* way for you to avoid or get out of the sexual abuse, then do you think God would consider it a sin?"

I think before speaking. God, I know, isn't to be trifled with.

"Well, God loves me and doesn't want me to be sexually abused," I process aloud. "It wouldn't make sense for Him to blame me for lying to get out of something like sexual abuse. Okay, I'm choosing no. I mean, no, I don't think God would consider it a sin if I lied about it not being my turn."

Maureen waits for me to finish writing.

"I bet I've asked forgiveness for that lie at least a thousand times," I add.

"Liz, remember when you told me you never tried to stop the abuse? Do you think that by saying it wasn't your turn, you *were* trying to stop it?"

My eyes widen in surprise, and I feel as if I've won a little lottery.

"I did try to stop it!" I say incredulously. "By saying 'not my turn,' I tried to stop him, just like Em and Sarah did."

"I'm going to throw out something else, Liz. What if saying it wasn't your turn wasn't a lie?"

I shake my head at her, unclear.

"Could we say it should never have been your turn?" she asks.

In my chair, I place my right hand over my mouth. "Maybe it was never my turn?" vibrates between my lips and through my fingers. My ears hear the question and my heart knows the answer. "It was never my turn," I whisper, savoring this truth. "It should've *never* been my turn." A new, lighter air fills my lungs.

"Can we do another?" I ask.

Maureen nods.

"Okay. I've been lying to Dad so I don't have to see him. He's always asking me to come over, but I tell him I have to work a double shift, when I don't."

"What are you feeling when he invites you over?" she asks.

"Jittery. Jumpy. I stutter a lot when I know I'm going to see him."

"Does *unsafe* fit? When you're with him, are you feeling not safe?" she asks.

"Yes, it fits," I reply, acknowledging that I like myself more after answering Maureen's questions.

"So by lying, you are able to stay away from your father and feel safe?"

"Yes," I confirm. "So, it's like the 'not my turn' lie. If the lie helps me stay safe, Jesus gets that. I won't go to hell for trying to stay safe."

I begin writing:

Two Steps to Understand Lying
Step 1—Ask what you're feeling.
Step 2—Ask what you are getting from lying. If it's good (keeping your-self safe), relax; Jesus will go to bat for you.

"So when I'm lying to keep myself safe, I can let it go. This is better than seeing myself as a bad seed with a long, pathological history of lying."

"Liz, the crux of why you want to resolve this issue is because you care about truth as it relates to trust. The conflict arose when you realized that to survive in your family, your only choice was to lie. You were lying to survive."

"And I got good at it. Like anything you practice, you get good at it."

"Yes, you got good at surviving."

"So I'm not a bad seed, then, either."

"Do you know where this 'bad seed' idea comes from?"

"I think I do. As a kid, my only choice was to lie, so I lied a lot. Then I ended up worrying that I was a bad seed because I lied so much, when I was just trying to stop the sexual abuse."

"A huge catch-22," Maureen confirms. "So lying to avoid seeing your dad—how does that sit with you now?"

"Much more comfortably. I'm not saying it is okay to lie, but if I have to choose between lying and keeping myself safe, I can choose to lie, at least for now."

"You've needed to lie to keep yourself safe in your family, and even then you weren't safe," Maureen affirms.

"No, back then I wasn't able to stay safe. But now I can. And I know, I *believe*, God wants me to be safe. Okay, one more?"

She nods.

"If I look at the grocery bill lie I told Matt...let's see here." I pause, reviewing my notes as I speak. "I lied because I felt guilty that I went over the budget."

"What happens when you go over the budget?" she asks.

"Nothing. So here there's no reason to lie. And because I want to be trustworthy, when I go home today, I'll tell Matt I lied about going over the budget."

"How do you think he'll respond?"

"He won't care. He eats as much junk food as me."

Maureen chuckles.

I look at the clock and see I have just five minutes left.

"This isn't on my list, but today, I mean, realizing today it was never my turn is *huge*. Shouldn't I be angry at Dad? Why do I only feel anger toward Mom?"

"What do you feel toward your father?"

"For my whole life, I've felt sorry for him…but now I don't know. Emptiness? Indifference? I'm not sure." I shrug.

"Feelings are never right or wrong. They just are. They may change or stay the same, but there's nothing wrong with wondering why you feel how you feel."

I nod. "That helps, about the lying."

"I'm glad, Liz." She tears off my copy of her notes and smiles. "I'm glad it helps."

Exiting Maureen's office, I make my way to my car. I scour my mind for other lies so I can practice my new two-step program. Still parked in Maureen's parking lot, I consider my lying about aspirin.

I lie to Matt about how much aspirin I take. I tell him I take two per day when I really take between six and eight.

What am I feeling when I tell the aspirin lie?

Fear. Fear because I know I need aspirin to survive.

And what am I getting from telling the lie?

I'm keeping the headaches away. The word *headache* provokes a particular kind of fear I cannot bear. At the first inkling of head pain, I immediately eliminate it. Even if it's not a pain, any sensation near my head is chased off by some water and two aspirin.

I have a bottle of aspirin in my car, one in my purse, and one in my desk. I always wear pants with pockets so I can keep two tablets with me at all times. If forced to choose between food and aspirin, I would definitely choose aspirin.

The only headaches I'm unable to ward off are the ones I awaken with. But I keep aspirin and a glass of water right near my bed so I'm always prepared. Always.

And when a headache goes away? I'm overcome with torrential relief, so grateful that I praise God for creating the person who invented aspirin.

I realize this lie is more complex. I should've discussed this lie with Maureen.

In the quietness of my car, I focus and go back to the second step: what am I getting by lying about the aspirin?

It dawns on me. It is relief I am seeking, the relief I felt each time his migraine would go away. I lie to keep my aspirin because aspirin gives me the power to make headaches go away. I can't have headaches in my life again. It would be the end of me.

I realize I will never give up that kind of power.

Not even for Matt.

SEVENTEEN

Slumber Party

Birthday privileges at the Luther household included choosing her favorite meal for dinner and exemptions from all chores—no housework, no dishes, and no back rubs. Those were the birthday rules.

The dining room table boasted a fried chicken feast with all the trimmings when Elizabeth's friends, five girls from the Church of Christ, arrived. Later, when the litter of birthday trimmings was disposed of and the devil's food cake had been devoured, it was slumber party time.

Sheets and blankets soon draped the oversized dining room table, cloaking an array of pillows, sleeping bags, chips, and soda.

Whispered giggles accompanied the typical Luther nighttime bustle. As the other children were put to bed, the volume outside the girls' fort gradually quieted until only one pair of footsteps padded about the house.

"Girls?" began Elizabeth's mother, parting the sheets that formed the makeshift door.

"Yes, Mrs. Luther," answered the girls in sing-song voices.

Elizabeth's mother laughed aloud as six heads with wide eyes peered up at her.

"Remember," she began, toning down her smile, "stay up as late as you like, but keep the noise down, okay?"

Heads nodded, and Elizabeth's mother stood.

"Thanks, Mom," Elizabeth called out.

"You're welcome," she replied. "Have fun."

The room darkened as her mother turned off the lights, one by one. Elizabeth parted the sheet, and with the help of the moon's light, saw her mom approaching the stairwell that led to her bedroom.

At last, everyone was in bed.

"Truth or Dare?" Margie whispered.

"I'm in," said Naomi, among a chorus of whispered agreements.

"Who goes first?" Margie asked.

"Liz. It's her birthday," said Naomi.

"Margie can go first," Liz offered. "It was her idea."

All eyes turned upon Margie.

"Have you ever seen?" Margie hesitated. "Have you ever seen a—"

"Ever seen a what?" Naomi hissed.

"A penis!" Margie whispered, raising her eyebrows.

Naomi's eyes bulged, and everyone buried their faces in their pillows resulting in a muffled, muted explosive laughter filled the tiny fort. Everyone except Elizabeth.

Of course she'd seen a penis.

"Wait!" whispered Terrie. "We need to take a vow of secrecy." Reaching under her pillow for her Bible, she placed it in the middle of the circle.

"Put your hand on mine," she directed, placing her hand on the Bible first. "Repeat after me. Nothing said here will *ever* be repeated. Swear to God, hope to die, stick a needle in my eye."

All hands followed suit, and everyone murmured in unison.

"Remember, you'll go to hell if you tell," she added.

Heads nodded. Of course they would.

"It looks like a hot dog," said Naomi.

Everyone stared at her, dumbfounded.

"Well, it does." She shrugged. "My mom says it's nothing to be ashamed of, either. It's how God made a man. None of us could have babies if it weren't for a penis."

Nothing to be ashamed of, Elizabeth considered. Eyeing her friend, she wondered if Naomi was *her* dad's favorite.

Pouring herself more soda and closing her eyes as the fizz speckled her nose, Elizabeth wondered what it would be like to stop worrying about not telling and just tell. After all, her friends were telling.

"I touched a penis," Terrie whispered, raising her eyebrows. "It was weird."

"What'd it look like?" Margie asked.

"I couldn't see it too good—it was dark. It was in the backseat of my boyfriend's car. It was kind of soft on the outside, like baby skin, but underneath the soft skin, it was stiff, stiffer than a hot dog," she finished.

Gaining confidence in her friend's disclosure, Elizabeth reminded herself they'd all taken an oath on God's Holy Word. Besides, everyone in her house was in bed. She'd seen her mother enter the stairwell with her own eyes.

Or had she?

Parting the blanket entrance with her left hand, the moon's glow illuminated the brown paneling two-thirds of the way down from the ceiling. The remaining lower third of the wall was black. As she allowed the makeshift door to close, she realized she hadn't heard the fourth stair step creak. She reasoned she could have missed it amid the whispering chatter.

Still uneasy, she parted wide the makeshift doorway a second time. Resisting the urge to hurry, she allowed her eyes to adjust to the darkness. Combing every inch of the floor and walls from top to bottom she paused, listening.

A slight aberration—was it a sniff?—leaped at her from the dark corner nearest the stairwell. Her eyes darted toward the disturbance, and although the moonlight could only partially illuminate the corner, Elizabeth was able to identify a crouching silhouette. Mom.

Her heart was beating through her chest as she allowed the makeshift door to close. Overcome with relief that she'd not revealed her secret, she praised God. Just as quickly, however, her stomach reeled as she replayed her friends' disclosures. Her mother would consider it her spiritual duty to inform respective parents of any improprieties.

Panicking, Liz feigned an elongated, too-loud yawn and stretched her arms out, then pushed upward, dislodging the dining room table leaf.

"Oops!" she whispered as the leaf clunked back into place. "Hey, I'm low on soda," she continued. "Anyone else want some?"

"I gotta use the bathroom," whispered Naomi.

Six bodies began scooting and shuffling around when an unexpected loud yawn from outside their encampment startled them. The subsequent flick of a light switch revealed six horrified faces in the now muted glow of the still-cloaked fort.

The girls looked at each other in dead silence, frozen in place. Everyone was holding their breath.

"Sorry to interrupt but I gotta use the bathroom," Liz's mother commented in a faux groggy voice, passing through the dining area on her way to the bathroom.

Seconds later the girls heard the bathroom door closing.

"Ya think she heard anything?" Terrie whispered desperately.

"No, she said she was sleeping," said Naomi. "She just had to pee. I gotta go, too. Come on, let's get some soda."

Replenishing their snack supply, Elizabeth heard her mother exit the bathroom and caught a glimpse of her as she passed the kitchen archway.

"Have fun," her mother whispered.

Elizabeth paused until she heard the telltale stair creak, and then, on her way back to the fort, she dropped a bag of chips near the entrance at the base of the stairs. Peering around the door-frame, she made certain no one was there.

Settling back into their fort, Naomi began.

"Where did we leave off?"

"Guys, I'm wiped out," Elizabeth announced.

"Come on," Naomi heaved a sigh. "You're only sixteen once."

"We have church tomorrow," Elizabeth attempted, "you guys should go to sleep, too."

"Party pooper," Naomi whispered.

As her friends continued playing Truth or Dare, Elizabeth closed her eyes and began her evening prayers. Culling through her day for any hint of sin, she asked God's forgiveness for those sins she didn't remember committing. She next prayed for each member of her family, except her mother.

Last, she begged Jesus to intervene on behalf of her friends, especially Terrie. She prayed her mother would consider choosing to keep their secrets safe.

The following morning, Elizabeth awoke to the telephone ringing and her mother's muffled voice. Rubbing her eyes to waken herself, she parted the makeshift door and looked toward the phone table. The phone was not there.

Crawling out from the fort, she followed the telephone cord and her mother's voice to the living room.

"Well," her mother murmured, "I know if it were my girl, you'd let me know. Sexual purity is so important at this age, at any age," she continued. Turning her head over her shoulder suspiciously, her mother paused at the sight of Elizabeth. "Well, the girls are getting up, so I guess I'd better let you go," she murmured, turning away from Elizabeth.

Twenty minutes later, Terrie's parents were knocking on the door. Terrie had to go home.

Later, at church, Terrie's father sat alone in the back row.

Elizabeth knew Terrie was home, likely still crying, maybe bruised from a beating. After the barn, Elizabeth had to stay home for at least a day or two so the welts would fade.

Elizabeth's heart burned in hatred for her mother. And then, an overwhelming sadness enveloped her. Terrie must think Elizabeth had told on her. She had not seen her mother eavesdropping, and there could be no other explanation. As the Lord's Supper was passed her way, she declined the unleavened bread and grape juice.

She was simply too unclean.

EIGHTEEN

Sadness

"I did your Little Girl homework assignment, but I'm not sure I did it right," I begin.

Maureen smiles. "There was no wrong way to do it, you know. How did it go?"

"Well, Matt was out of town. I put my sweats on, lit a candle, and sat on the couch. And she came to me, just like that." I snapped my fingers. "It wasn't hard at all. She looked like a little girl ghost—a foggy little spirit. I could see right through her. She just walked up and down the steps to her father's bedroom, back and forth, back and forth." I pause. "That was it. What do you make of it?"

"I think it's good that she came to you so readily. It's a great start," Maureen replies. "And I'd like you to do it again."

"I can do that." Looking up, I'm still holding my pen. "Can I go on to number two?"

"Sure, number two."

"I told Sarah I was in therapy."

Maureen raises her eyebrows. "She's the sister who works at the psychiatric hospital with you?"

"Yes. She asked who I was seeing, and I told her you. She already knew who you were. She met you once when she worked as a fill-in on the adult floor. She thinks it's a good idea."

"Why does she think it's good?"

"She liked how you talked to your clients, and how you talked about them during the team meetings. And because she knows me. I know I'm the oldest girl, but it's obvious I have more issues than Sarah ever had.

"Although I'm the oldest sister, I seem to have more, well, let's just say I have more issues than Sarah. We've talked about it though. I mean, I can be honest with her. We kind of agree that because she saw 'normal' at twelve and I saw it at sixteen, she kind of got a head start on what normal looked like. And Dad stopped with her when she confronted him at twelve; I never had that in me back then, so it just kept happening until I was removed at sixteen."

"That makes sense," Maureen confirmed.

"We also talked about Dad, too. How he's always said he doesn't remember what happened, and he didn't know who he was with. And Maureen? Sarah did the weirdest thing. She *laughed* at Dad's reasoning. I mean, she *laughed out loud*, like his explanation was ridiculous. She told me outright, she thinks Dad knew all along what he was doing. Lately, I've *considered* he might have known, but not enough to say it aloud to anyone. Well, except now, with you."

"Why do you think you're starting to consider your father might have known what he was doing?"

"Well, as Sarah pointed out, Dad spoke to me during the back rubs; he called me by name and told me I was his favorite. And I've always known that, but because he said he never knew who he was with in bed, I automatically believed him. I don't think it ever crossed my mind to disagree with him because I was always so afraid. Now that I'm not so afraid, I wonder about things on more of a cognitive level. I can examine things in my head, even question things, rather than just accepting them as fact because my father said them. If he didn't know who he was with, how could he call me by name?" I grab two tissues and wipe my eyes. "And don't mind these tears." I add. "I've been crying on and off like this all week since I talked to Sarah. Even called in sick yesterday because of it."

Maureen smiles reassuringly. "Liz, there's nothing wrong with crying; crying means you are making connections, and that's what healing is all about. So, considering your dad may have known what he was doing, what does that mean for you?"

"That it's my choice now. It's my choice to determine if he knew what he was doing or not. I never knew I had a choice. I never knew I had the right to think, to choose for myself."

"So you can choose for yourself."

"Yes, and this is going to sound strange, I know." My voice is starting to quiver. "But if it ends up, I mean, if I decide Dad knew what he was doing? I won't die."

"When you say you won't die, what do you mean?"

"As a kid, I was always terrified, to the point of death. I know it sounds melodramatic, but I swear, if I'd have disobeyed either of my parents when I was a kid and had died as a result of the up and coming discipline that always followed, I wouldn't have been surprised. I never expected to live to adulthood. I never knew how afraid I was—the depth of it, and all the faces of it. I know what three dimensional is, but I don't know what you call it when the dimensions of something include the outside, the inside, and the inner *core* of the faces. And there's another component to this: I wasn't just afraid of disobeying and the aftermath of the barn; I was afraid of losing Dad's love and most afraid of double shifts. Without Dad's love—and I know that sounds gross in a way—but without him, my mother was so abusive, I would've felt totally abandoned.

"And when I was scared all the time, there was no way I could think like this. Sorry, here I go again." I grab two more tissues and wonder if Maureen has to spend some of her income on tissues. *Should I bring in a box to replenish her supply?*

"Cry as much as you need, Liz. It sounds like the absence of fear, or at least a lesser amount of fear, is allowing you to think more clearly."

I blow my nose and toss the tissue in the wastebasket.

"Yes. And it's opened up this door of sadness at the same time. When I consider the absence of love in my childhood, and that my parents may not have loved me…" I shake my head. "I just start crying. I can be in my car, at the grocery store, in the shower. I try to let it in, the sadness part, a little at a time. But sometimes it comes upon me without warning. I keep reminding myself that the sadness won't last forever. It won't swallow me whole like I thought it would. I won't die from it."

"Realizing your parents didn't love you is good reason to feel sad," Maureen murmurs.

"My entire childhood was lost. It's like a death."

"And people grieve for death and loss. It's important to honor that, to grieve your lost childhood, to cry as much as you need."

My tears continue in the silence.

"Liz, are you doing okay?"

"Ya know? I am. I may not look like it on the outside, but on the inside? I'm pretty good. When I cry like this, it's like I'm taking a shower from the inside out. I feel a different kind of clean. In hindsight, when I think of all the years I've refused to cry and tried to outrun the sadness by working double shifts—I just delayed the healing process. I may have done a good job avoiding the pain by denying the truth. But by denying the truth, I've played a part in perpetuating the lie—the lie that there was nothing to be sad about."

NINETEEN

Coming of Age

April 1981, sixteen years old

Liz gaped at the bloodstained underwear within the confines of the girl's bathroom stall. So *this* was her period. Wrapping her sweater around her waist, she hurried to the main office.

"Pads are in the bathroom on the back of the stool," the secretary said, nodding at the sweater tied around Liz's waist and then motioning to the women's room. "You'll find paper bags for your soiled clothes and clean clothes on the top shelf. You should be able to find something that fits. No worries, I'll call your mom right away."

Liz turned and locked herself inside. She spied the pads stacked atop the toilet tank and opened a pink, rectangular wrapper. She examined the contents with curiosity: a quilted, white, oblong shape. Examining the other side of the pad, she noticed

105

the wax-paper covering. Peeling it away, she further discovered the pink, tacky glue lines.

Ingenious.

Pressing the tacky side to her clean underwear and donning her new pants, she washed her hands. Checking the cabinet above the sink, she found a stack of paper bags and placed her soiled clothing inside one. Closing the lid of the stool, she sat upon it and waited for her mother.

Her mother arrived within thirty minutes to sign Liz out. They exited the school in silence.

The ride home was quiet, uneventful except for a stop at the grocery store. Her mother returned with a midsized brown paper bag and tossed it upon the backseat floorboard. The contents spilled out: Kotex Maxi Pads.

Elizabeth, lying down in the backseat, pressed her right palm against her aching forehead. Closing her eyes, she tried ignoring the knotting in her stomach. Twenty minutes later, she awakened to the sound of turning gravel. Grateful to be home, she went straight to bed.

She awoke later to the sound of her brothers and sisters entering the back door from the afternoon bus ride home. Next, she heard the family car pull into the driveway. Dad was home.

Realizing the pad needed to be changed, she made her way to the bathroom, where the brown paper grocery bag sat beside the toilet.

From the bathroom she heard Dad's voice. Her parents were just outside the bathroom door.

"It's no big deal. Just tell her, Beck," he said.

"No," her mother whispered. "You know how modest I am. You do it."

"It's natural," he interjected.

"I can't," her mother whined. "I won't."

A moment later her father knocked on the bathroom door, opened it, and stepped just inside. Still holding his black lunch box, he smiled at Liz still on the toilet, underwear around her ankles.

"We gotta talk," he said. "Your mother won't do it, so I'll have to. Meet me upstairs in my bedroom."

He closed the door.

After washing her hands, she met him in his bedroom. He was lying on his bed, hands clasped behind his head.

"It's nothing to be ashamed of," he said. "You know that, right?"

She nodded.

"You know, this means you can have a baby now," he began, patting a spot on the bed, motioning for her to sit.

She wondered what headaches, stomachaches, and blood had to do with babies.

"It's simple how it works," he began. "So simple you'll now see why we didn't let you attend those so-called health courses in junior high. They talk about sex before marriage and other worldly influences you don't need to worry about. It's easy: you got these egg sacks in you, and after you're married, the sacks will get fertilized and make a baby. Get it?"

She nodded.

"Good. Now you know what intercourse is," he continued. "So you know to never let a man in the house. He could rape you."

"I know," she replied, reaching for her still cramping stomach.

"A woman neither," he said.

"A woman?"

"Yes, a woman," he continued, addressing her obvious doubt. "A woman could find the broom and shove the handle right up your crotch."

She felt nauseated.

"Men will want to touch you, of course. That's natural. God made us that way. Once they get started, they can't stop. It's your job to say no. Any woman who doesn't say no is what the Bible calls a harlot, a whore."

Elizabeth felt very small.

"It's common sense. When two people have intercourse, who gets pregnant? It isn't the man. Getting pregnant is God's way of saying the woman is responsible for saying no; and if she doesn't, it's her fault and there will be consequences. There aren't any consequences for men having sex 'cause God knows men can't help it.

"Now the world will tell you it's okay to have sex before marriage. Take college women, they always have sex before marriage. That's why you'll never go to college, because no man will marry you. No man wants a whore for a wife."

She nodded.

"Good. One more thing," he said. "These days colored men like white women, especially blondes like you. You know God forbids mixing races."

Perplexed but wanting to go back to bed, she hesitated, then asked, "Old or New Testament?"

"Hmm, the verse where God talks about a cow not mating with a pig."

"What?" Unable to mask her annoyance, she checked her tone. Of course cows and pigs couldn't mate, but a brown pig and a pink pig could mate. Their own pigs were different colors and *had* mated.

"It's in there," he insisted. "People who mix up races are going against nature, and since God created nature, they're going against God."

She remembered Genesis: *And God saw everything that He had made, and behold, it was good.* Her fear of God exceeded her fear of her father, and she knew if she agreed with her father, she was in essence critiquing God's varied workmanship and questioning His competence. She remained silent.

"Okay then, so no more questions?" Dad asked.

She shook her head no.

"Good." He sighed, standing up. "I'm starving. Let's eat."

TWENTY

Salisbury Steak

Entering my haven, I open my notebook.

"I wrote s-s-something," I say, retrieving the folded, lined notebook paper and extending it to Maureen.

She accepts the paper and creases it open upon her clipboard.

"Salisbury steak?" she muses, wrinkling her brow.

"That's the t-title," I stammer. "My m-mom made the best Salisbury steak."

"Do you want me to read it aloud?"

I nod.

Maureen clears her throat and takes a sip of water.

"Salisbury Steak," she begins in a soft, clear voice. "My mom made the best Salisbury steak in the world, but she was the worst mom for me. As of late, when I am alone, I am feeling motherless."

110

Maureen pauses and takes a sip of water.

"It is not a desperate 'I need a mother right now,' emotion. I don't need a mother to hug me, kiss my forehead, or tousle my hair this instant. What I long for is a caring memory to go over in my mind and feel in my heart; a moment in time when I can grasp a remembrance that she used to hug me; that she used to kiss me. That she was, in some way, fond of me."

I inhale sharply at my own words.

Maureen continues reading: "It is a mystery why longing for such a memory weighs so heavily in its importance to me right now. It is an inconvenient desire.

"In the past I have not needed a mother; have not wanted a mother. In fact, in my own words, 'if that's a mother [my mother], then I don't want one.'

"But now, the adult in me sees how important it is to provide a child with love. Or maybe it's the child in me who yearns for what I never had—and at times pretended to have—because I was unable to acknowledge, much less accept, that I was not cared for.

"I cannot help but wonder, was I somehow unlovable or somehow made unlovable?"

Maureen takes another drink of water and then reads on. "I can only presume that, if I knew then what I am safely able to know now, as a child I would have felt as sad, empty, and defiled as I feel right now. And perhaps a little girl couldn't have endured such a feeling."

Maureen refolds the paper to its original form, extending it toward me. "That was powerful."

"I didn't cry when I wrote it," I said, wiping my eyes.

"Remember, crying—the sadness—is so important for healing."

I exhale and want to move on. "Number two?" I ask.

"Okay, number two."

"I did the Little Girl homework again. The first time I did it, she was an innocuous little ghost, kind of a spirit-girl going up and down the stairs. But she's different now."

"Different?" Maureen asks.

"Like a guest you don't mind at first. Then, as you get to know her, you realize you don't like her."

Maureen waits.

"She's gross. She disgusting. She's a liar. I hate her. I feel hate when I look at her."

"Liz, this is different from how you felt about her last time."

"Yes, and it's because this time as I watched her go up the steps, I knew that *she knew* what was going to happen. I followed her into his bed, and I saw her face. She was smiling," I lower my voice. "She was smiling."

"Why do you think she was smiling?" Maureen asks.

The words drip from my lips with disdain. "B-b-because she's a pathetic little slut who knew what she was doing. She can't fool me."

"And when you say, 'she can't fool me,' what do you mean by that?"

"She knew what was going to happen, and she says she didn't like it. So she shouldn't have been smiling," I accuse. "She must have liked it. You don't smile if you hate something."

"Liz, is there any other reason she could be smiling?"

Hesitating, I close my eyes and see her in bed with him. She is so little!

"While she w-was obeying him, she'd peek and see him watching her." I begin. "She was afraid he'd see she didn't like it. She had to please him, and it would hurt him if he knew she hated it. He said his headache was so bad—the pain was so bad—he could die. And she believed him when he said that."

"So she was pleasing him and didn't want to hurt him."

God, I am so dirty.

"Dirty?" Maureen asks.

I look at her and realize I spoke this thought aloud.

"What I did *was* dirty."

"Which part was dirty, the obeying part or the pleasing part?"

I am concentrating so hard I feel my head will explode.

"If by mopping the floor well he was pleased, that wouldn't be wrong. But touching each other to please is wrong."

"You called it 'touching each other'?"

I nod.

"Who was the adult?" she asks.

"Him," I say.

"On the children's unit at the hospital, who's in charge?" Maureen asks.

"The adult, so me."

"So the kids aren't in charge. Why?"

"The kids aren't capable of being in charge," I answer.

These words sit on my skin and dance.

"Yes, Liz. They're children. And who has the power on the unit, the kids or the adults?"

"The adults," I answer, seeing the connection. "I'm the one responsible because I have the power."

"You're right, Liz. The adults are in charge because they have the power. And children want to please adults."

"And kids believe adults, too," I add.

"Children should be able to believe adults, Liz."

"Yes. They should. And, Maureen? When he said I was his favorite? I believed him. And I wanted to stay his favorite, so I obeyed him. So he would keep on loving me."

"Do you think there's anything shameful about wanting to be loved by a parent?"

"I know in my head there's nothing shameful about wanting to please or be loved by a parent. But then why, in here"—I point to my constricting chest—"in here I feel so ashamed?"

Maureen cocks her head and turns her right hand palm-side up, beckoning me to answer my own question.

My head at odds with my emotions, I begin. "If fatherly love and sexual touching are wrong, then my father did not love me. And fatherly love without sexual touching—is *that* real love then? It's distorted. I *feel* distorted. I feel abnormal."

"Yes and no. Your father did distort love for you, but you are not abnormal. Your feelings are normal for your life experience. Know inside your head that you are normal to feel how you're feeling right now."

"You know what I wish?" I ask, tapping my fingers on my breast. "I wish I could feel clean, in here."

"It's normal for you to not feel clean. And Liz? I'm wondering something. Do you think this has anything to do with you feeling defiled?"

"Hmm?" I ask, unsure of her question.

"You said something about feeling defiled in your essay." She reaches for my paper and opens it. "Here, right here: 'If I knew then what I am safely able to know now, as a child I would have felt as sad, empty, and defiled as I feel right now.'"

"I'd say it has everything to do with it. All those years, Maureen! Why was I silent for so many years?"

"You were silent because it's all you were allowed to be."

"Silence and obedience are intertwined, but they are not the same thing. I mean, to do anything except be silent would've been disobedient. And disobedience wasn't allowed. So I was stuck between a rock and a hard place. Wait!" A kaleidoscope of hope whirls around me. "If being obedient wasn't wrong, because I obeyed Dad in bed and obedience was expected, then"—I hesitate—"does this mean I'm not a slut?"

Maureen pauses, and I think she wants me to answer my own question. The thing is, I was called a slut so often by Mom, to consider anything else would be like saying land was water. Holding my breath I silently plead for Maureen to answer the question for me, just for today, just this once. I need to hear what it sounds like.

"Liz," Maureen's voice rings out bold and sure, piercing the chaos. "You are not a slut. You never were."

My whisper seems to take wing with each word that leaves my mouth. "I am not a slut." I smile a little, and a soft voice fills the room. It is my voice, and it is more than a whisper. "I see it now. I was obedient; never, never a slut."

Maureen extends her hand and I shake it.

I think this is what joy must feel like.

TWENTY-ONE

Coming Home

Her first weekend away from home was coming to a close, and she was already formulating a plan to extend her vacation.

She had gone to Cedar Point (for free!) with a family from church. In exchange for helping Doug and JoAnne take care of their three young children, she ate fast food, slept in a hotel, and rode as many rides as she pleased. She had never done so little, received so much, slept so well, or felt so appreciated.

They pulled into Doug and JoAnne's driveway, and Elizabeth began unpacking the car. She planned to start a load of laundry, then offer to give Mary, the baby, her bath. Hopefully, nighttime would creep up on them, and it would be too late to take her home.

Tumbling out of the car, Luke and Katie ran to their grandparents, who were awaiting their arrival in the driveway. Titus and Olivia, who lived next door, were the longest-standing members of the local Church of Christ. Titus's brother, Tom, had led Elizabeth's dad to the Lord.

Carrying a suitcase inside the house along with her paper grocery bag filled with her own belongings, Elizabeth let the wooden screen door thump closed behind her. Placing her bag on the kitchen table, she noticed no one followed her. A squeal of laughter filtered through the screen door, and peering outside, she saw the children playing on the swing set as the adults visited in the driveway.

Taking the toiletries suitcase to the bathroom and setting it upon the marble countertop, she heard the kitchen door creak open. She padded down the carpeted hallway and stopped in the doorway.

Four adults stood around the kitchen table. Doug, Titus, and Olivia were looking at the floor. JoAnne was looking at Elizabeth.

"'Lizabeth," said JoAnne, leading her out of the kitchen toward the living room. Let's go sit on the sofa for a minute."

"Who d-died?" Elizabeth whispered as she obeyed. She wondered if God had allowed her mother to be killed.

"No one died," JoAnne murmured.

"Then what?" she asked, her eyes darting from JoAnne and Olivia on either side of her and then to Titus and Doug standing on the carpet near the sofa.

Titus spoke next.

"Your sisters, Emma and Sarah—they told the police about your dad."

Elizabeth paused. "Told what?"

An uncomfortable silence choked the air.

"About the touching," whispered Olivia.

Trembling, Elizabeth shook her head in disbelief. She'd never told anyone about the backrubs. Did her sisters know her secret?

"Where's my d-d-dad?" she asked panicking.

"On his way to jail," Titus replied.

Elizabeth waited for the universe to reset. From outside, musical squeals of childhood poked at her ears as the summer breeze annoyed the white and blue checkered curtains in the window.

She lowered her eyes to the carpet then covered her face with both hands. She knew what they were thinking. She was a whore.

"Liz, it's okay. He can't hurt you anymore," said JoAnne.

From a distance, a humming engine coursed along the gravel road. The dull noise grew until a roaring engine blared into the driveway, spewing gravel.

Her heart constricting, she knew it was her mother.

Titus and Doug glanced at one another, then exited via the screen door.

Olivia joined Elizabeth and JoAnne on the couch, and Elizabeth heard men's voices rise and lower on the Michigan wind.

Todd?

It *was* Todd; first in the doorway, then in the kitchen. He stopped at the sight of Elizabeth sitting between JoAnne and Olivia.

"Liz, let's go," he commanded.

"Todd," Doug spoke, coming from behind with Titus in tow. "Calm down; you can't drive like this."

"Liz, the cops are at the house, and they want your ass," Todd demanded.

Elizabeth froze. Why would the police want her ass?

"We'll take her," said JoAnne.

Elizabeth paused.

"No," Todd said defiantly, "I gave 'em my word. I'm taking her."

No one moved, so Elizabeth rose.

JoAnne stood, turning her face toward Elizabeth's ear.

"Call us anytime," she whispered. "We love you."

Willing her feet forward, she passed Todd, snatching her paper bag from the kitchen table.

Outside she felt Todd's hand on her back as he tried to hurry her.

"Don't!" she snarled, turning on him. "Don't *ever* touch me again!"

Withdrawing both of his hands, he held them high in the air. "God, Liz! Okay," he said, lowering his voice.

She climbed into the front passenger's seat as Todd made his way into the driver's seat.

"So, you heard what Emma's done?" Todd seethed.

She was silent.

"Doug said they told you. Did they?" he asked, spinning out the tires as he backed out.

She remained silent.

"Guess I'll tell you myself, then. Emma told some church people that Dad's been messing around with her. The church people called the cops. Everything's gone to hell."

"Huh?" Elizabeth whispered, eyes widening in disbelief.

"I know," he seethed, slamming his palm on the steering wheel and gaining speed, dust spewing in his wake. "The cops don't know Emma lies. And Sarah's not helping, either."

"Sarah?" Elizabeth yelped, gasping in confusion.

"Yeah, Sarah decided to go along with Emma's little story." He sneered, still gaining speed on the gravel road. "I can set Sarah straight once I talk to her, but the cops won't let me near her."

The lone stop sign at Clinton Trail appeared in the distance. As Todd tapped his brakes, an odd waggling of the car unnerved her. As if careening across marbles, the car began fishtailing wildly from one side of the road to the other.

"Hang on!" Todd shouted and the two lurched forward, their hands bracing against the dashboard as the car slammed to a thunderous stop.

She turned toward him, glaring.

He did not look at her.

Placing his hands back on the wheel, he accelerated more slowly this time, turning right onto the rural highway.

"Liz," he paused, his voice softening, "I need to know something."

His foreign, kind tone placed her on high alert. She turned toward him, and brother and sister locked eyes. She was nauseated at his obvious and utter insincerity. Raising her eyebrows, she stared at him hatefully, unblinking.

Looking away he cleared his throat.

"I already know the answer," he said, his familiar air of superiority returning. "But I'm asking you anyway, and I'm only asking once, so you better tell me the truth."

Staring straight ahead, she could not fathom his audacity. Who did he think he was asking anything of her? He was the enemy.

"Were you and Dad messing around?" he asked.

Indignant, she scoffed at the notion of betraying her father, and of all people, to betray him to Todd? Never.

"Well?" he shouted.

Shaking her head once, she kept her eyes on the road ahead.

"I knew it," he spat. "Make sure you—"

"Where are Em and Sarah?"

"Some foster home. But Uncle Jeff and Aunt Sheila are coming from Colorado to get them. Something about it's better to keep the kids with relatives. But Liz, you have to tell the cops that nothing—"

"Where's Dad?" she asked, interrupting him again.

"At home, with the cops," he replied.

Relieved her father wasn't on his way to jail as Titus had reported, she continued. "And the other kids?"

"Home," he replied.

She fell silent.

"Mom's home, too," he added. "And when you get home, you're supposed to meet her in the bathroom. Don't talk to anyone till you see her."

As they eased over the final hill and their house came into view, she was stunned at the four police cars dotting each side of the house. Todd brought the car to a stop in the driveway, and her stomach rolled as uniformed officers lingered near the doors and windows of her home.

"Remember, Mom's in the bathroom. Don't forget to—"

Opening the car door she cut him off, slamming the door shut behind her. Hugging her paper bag, she crossed the lawn, but slowed upon noticing a tall police officer standing just inside the back door. He was wearing a short-sleeved, dark blue uniform, and a gun hung from his black, thick belt. She would have to make it past him to get to the bathroom.

The policeman likewise noticed her and poked his head out of the doorway, ducking to avoid hitting his head on the top of the doorframe. He reached for a black walkie-talkie and his lips began moving. Her peripheral vision noted two male uniforms starting toward her.

Trying not to panic, she made her way to the back door, hesitating as she came upon the police officer who stood at least six feet tall.

He acknowledged her with a head nod; she nodded back as she rushed for the bathroom door. Fumbling for the doorknob, she opened the door and slid inside, inadvertently slamming the door closed. Tossing her paper bag to the floor, she leaned against the bathroom door, exhaling in relief.

A small shuffling interrupted her reprieve.

Opening her eyes and looking toward the darkened corner, she saw her mother coursing toward her like a snake.

TWENTY-TWO

Patterns

"Okay, I don't think I'm reading into this." I shift in my pink chair. "But I want to see what you think. Back in March, Dad had a mild heart attack and was in the hospital a few days. I visited him and brought him some pictures I'd taken at Christmas. I told him if he liked them, I'd make reprints.

"After he was released from the hospital, I called to check on him and asked if he'd liked any of the pictures. He said he liked them, but he'd misplaced them.

"Then Florence, Dad's wife, had a birthday. I stopped by their house to leave her some flowers. No one was home, so I used my key to get in and left the flowers on the kitchen counter. As I stood in the kitchen, I noticed a framed collage of the pictures I'd loaned

123

Dad sitting on top of their entertainment center. Annoyed, I took them back.

"The next night Dad called me with this eerie tone in his voice. He said, 'I'm not mentioning names, but someone stole some things from our home, and we'd like them back.'

"I asked if he'd called the police, and he said no. Then he said something about pictures being priceless. I asked, 'Are you talking about my pictures?' and he said, 'No, I'm talking about *my* pictures.'

"I reminded him I'd loaned him the pictures while he was in the hospital. Do you know what he said? 'For Christ sake, Lizzie, I'd just had a heart attack! I was in so much pain and on so much medicine, I don't remember who I was talking to, much less what they said!'"

Maureen's eyebrows raise and do not lower.

"That's *exactly* like the back rubs," I say incredulously. "It's a pattern—it's *evidence*."

"Evidence that proves—"

"That he's capable of lying—lying like I'm an idiot. This wasn't something that happened ten years ago and I could've gotten confused. I knew the truth, and I wasn't going to deny the truth for him. Then I said I didn't appreciate him calling me a thief. He said, 'I never called you a thief. I just said you took something without permission.' I told him if I left my purse on his couch, I wouldn't need his permission to take it because it was *mine*. And it wasn't hard speaking to him the way I did because I *knew* my truth was real. I felt so powerful!"

"You're choosing to believe in your truth."

"Yes I am," I reply.

"And you do have power," Maureen confirms. "You stood up to him."

Leaning back in my chair, I smile at this newer version of me. I realize the next item on my list also validates another transformation.

"Okay, second thing: at work a guy put his hand on my leg and started rubbing my thigh. In the beginning I froze, like usual. Then, when I remembered I was supposed to do something different, I couldn't remember the plan we'd talked about earlier. Remember, the one where I'd say no?"

"I remember," she says, nodding.

"So, you know what I did? I stood up—shaking like a leaf, by the way—but I still stood up and pushed that man's hand right off my thigh. Then I walked down the hall and into the staff bathroom."

"That's big for you." Maureen replies. She picks up her pen and jots something down.

"And when I got to the bathroom and looked in the mirror? I was surprised to see me in there, in the mirror, all in one piece. It took me a few minutes to calm down. Then I realized I'd made it stop. Me! What I've been working on in this little room is spilling out into my world!" I laugh aloud.

Who is this girl in the pink chair? I wonder.

"An empowering, new experience for you," Maureen replies, the corners of her mouth turning upward in a smile.

"It was new, and I thought it would be so hard to make it stop, but it wasn't. The hardest part was remembering to do something *different*."

"It sounds like you tried something new and it worked. You kept yourself safe."

"Yes, I can depend on me to keep myself safe," I say, still smiling.

"Yes, you can," she replies. "Usually. But there are times that are out of anyone's control."

I nod, knowing she is quite right about that.

"Oh, Liz, I've been meaning to ask you something and keep forgetting. Do you have any pictures of yourself when you were a child, say in your elementary years?"

"I don't, but Rachel is still talking to Mom. I bet she could get some for me."

"That would be great. Could you bring the pictures to therapy some time?"

"Sure," I reply. "Oh, last thing," I interject, seeing we have just two minutes left. "Did you catch that article in the paper about the woman who is suing her father for sexually abusing her when she was a child?"

"I did," Maureen replies. "What did you think of that?"

"I think that's pretty courageous."

"That would take courage," Maureen affirms.

"One day I'd like to meet her," I say as I stand.

"You would?"

"Yes. I'd like to tell her how brave she is and thank her for her example of bravery."

Maureen tears off my copy of her notes. "You could, Liz. And you could also look in the mirror and thank yourself for the same thing."

TWENTY-THREE

Bargain

Index finger pressed over her lips, she drew close to Elizabeth, revealing a gray complexion, puffy, red eyes, and lips trembling to the point of grimacing.

Aghast at her mother's appearance, Elizabeth stepped away from her, inadvertently distancing herself from the door.

Her mother grasped the knob, locking them in.

As her mother reached for her, a bewildered Elizabeth took another step backward, unsure of what Mom's intentions were. Her mother then hugged her, even as Elizabeth flinched in her grasp then pulled away.

"Thank God you're home," Mom whispered, withdrawing her shaking hands. "You know what'll happen if you tell the truth about your father. He'll go to prison for fifteen years. He'll be raped and sleep on a cement floor. He'll eat bread and water."

Elizabeth froze in fear; she could never survive her mother without her father.

"And your sisters. Since Emma's told these lies about your father, they're in a foster home, maybe being beaten or raped." Her voice faded.

A horrific tempest whirled around Elizabeth as she considered her father and sisters raped.

"Do you love your dad?" Mom began, reaching again for Liz.

She shoved Mom away, agitated. "*Stop* trying to touch me!" she hissed.

"Okay, okay," her mother whimpered, wrapping her arms around herself. "I said, do you love your father?"

"Y-yes. B-But if I lie, I'm going to hell," Elizabeth whispered.

Mom shook her head vehemently. "No, the lie will go on my head. Your job is to obey."

"So, if you were me—" Elizabeth paused, wanting to be sure the potential penalty of hell was reserved solely for her mother. "If you w-were me, you'd lie? And since I'm obeying you, I won't go to hell?"

"Of course, that's right from the Bible. Ephesians—"

"I know the v-verse," Elizabeth interrupted. "But if you were me—"

"I'd lie—the same way I lied when it happened with me and my dad."

Elizabeth winced, struggling to imagine her mom as anyone's favorite.

"So y-you l-lied for Grandpa? He t-t-touched you?" she whispered incredulously.

Mom nodded pitifully. "I loved my daddy, so I lied for him. What daughter wouldn't?"

Reeling from Mom's disclosure, Elizabeth closed her eyes and shook her head back and forth. "Wait—what about Em—and Sarah?"

"Why are you changing the subject?" Mom began. "We were talking about—"

"God, Mom!" Elizabeth hissed in exasperation. "Who will take care of them? They're all alone!"

"Okay, keep your voice down," Mom pled. "Of course I'm worried about them. They're my flesh and blood. And now that I'm the legal guardian of all you kids, not your dad, what I say goes. If you lie, I can make sure you go with Emma and Sarah."

"You can?"

"Because of Emma's lies, your dad has no rights to any of you. It's just us girls now." Mom's voice cracked as she covered her face with both hands. "We've got to stick together."

"So if I lie, I'll go with the girls?" Elizabeth clarified.

"Yes," Mom assured.

"Todd said that Uncle Jeff's coming, and Em and Sarah might go with him and Aunt Sheila. If they do, can I still go with them?"

"Yes," said her mother. "You know I've always hated my brother, so it's best you go along to watch over the girls."

"So, if I lie, I g-g-go with Em and Sarah, *today*. You promise."

"Promise," Mom replied, placing her hand upon her heart.

"Swear on your life," Elizabeth pressed.

"I swear on my life."

"Okay," Elizabeth replied.

There was a brief pause.

"Now you know the cops will ask you questions," Mom began.

Liz's stomach muscles knotted. "What do I say?" she whispered.

"Just say Em lies, that's the truth anyway. She's always lied," Mom replied.

"What about Sarah?"

"Say she just went along with Emma's story." Mom shrugged.

"What about the back rubs?" Elizabeth continued.

Mom paused. "You could always say you don't remember," she reasoned. "It's not like you can say the exact day and hour you gave him a back rub."

Elizabeth realized this was true.

"So we have a deal then?" Mom asked.

"If I lie, I go with Em and Sarah today, no matter what. You swear it." Elizabeth restated.

"On God's honor," Mom vowed.

Elizabeth nodded.

"Good. Okay then, the cops are waiting to question you, so you better go. I'll hide in here for a bit so no one knows we were together."

Elizabeth's mother unlocked the door, stood behind it, and waved Elizabeth out.

Walking into the toy room, Elizabeth found herself facing the same officer she'd passed earlier. He smiled, and she smiled back, inwardly dubbing him the Toy Room Police Officer.

A fluttering movement from the picture window caught her eye. Turning, she saw Dad with a white pillowcase draped over his head. His hands were behind his back and fastened together with handcuffs. Two officers led him to a black-and-white police car and guided him into the backseat.

Her heart racing, Elizabeth knew she must hurry and tell the lie. She must save her father before it was too late.

A man in a gray suit began walking toward the house.

"Detective," announced the Toy Room Officer through the open doorway. "Our young lady is in here."

Elizabeth watched as the man entered and both men shook hands. Amid their greeting, Elizabeth spied a black revolver strapped beneath the detective's gray suit coat.

The Toy Room Officer nodded at Elizabeth, then assumed his bodyguard stance.

The detective turned toward her. "Elizabeth?" he asked kindly.

She nodded at him, thinking he was the same age as her father.

"I'm Detective Sims. Can we talk in my car?"

"Oh no, you don't!" Mom screeched, bolting from the bathroom.

Startled, Elizabeth jumped as the Toy Room Officer took two large steps, barricading Elizabeth from her mother.

"Ma'am!" he commanded.

"Don't you 'ma'am' me!" Her mother sneered, looking up at the officer. "I know my rights. She's *my* daughter, a minor! You don't have *my* permission to question her! Who knows what you perverts will do to her?"

"Whoa!" said the Toy Room Officer in the deepest, loudest voice Elizabeth had ever heard. Eye level with his biceps, Elizabeth watched the veins in his muscles spring into deep blue, palpable ridges. She felt her right hand move upward and realized it would be inappropriate to touch his veins. She lowered her hand.

"Mrs. Luther," he ordered, "Detective Sims is going to question Elizabeth in his car, in your driveway, in plain sight. He doesn't need your permission to question her under these circumstances. The question is, do you want her questioned here or down at the station?"

Cowering beneath his gaze, Mom fell silent.

In the quietness, Detective Sims glanced at Elizabeth then extended his arm in invitation toward the door. Her feet began moving, and he walked alongside her, guiding her toward the dark sedan parked behind the police car her father was in. He opened the front passenger's door, and she slid in.

Directly in front of her, through the rear window of the police car, she saw a small, flag-like section of the white pillowcase rustle above the top of the backseat.

Was Dad trying to signal her?

Narrowing her eyes in concentration, she looked down and wondered what Dad could be trying to tell her. She noticed now the console, the long black barrel of a rifle bolted into it between the driver's and passenger's seat.

The detective walked around the front of the sedan and entered on the driver's side. Liz wondered why he needed a handgun and a rifle if he only wanted to ask her some questions.

He placed his arm behind her seat, upon the shoulder rest above her head, and she noticed his five o'clock shadow. He smiled.

Will he kiss me?

He leaned forward, and she froze, closing her eyes, holding her breath. She felt nothing, and when she heard his hands fumbling near the console, she opened her eyes to see him holding a small black box. His lips were moving, and her eyes darted between his mouth and the shifting white pillowcase in the police car ahead of them.

She wondered if the detective could check on her father. He might have a migraine and need his pills.

The barn loomed in front of her father's police car, while to her left, through the long green fronds of the weeping willow, her mother stood in the doorway, arms folded beneath her breasts.

The white pillowcase moved again, and Elizabeth began fidgeting, now certain her father was trying to send her a message. But what?

Turning toward the detective, she wondered if he thought her a whore. Or maybe he had a favorite daughter? If he did, then he might understand.

Writing on some paper strapped to a clipboard, the detective looked at her expectantly. Elizabeth realized he had asked her a question.

"I d-d-don't remember," she stammered.

He paused, furrowing his brow as if confused.

"Emma lies," she offered.

His lips were moving again, and as Elizabeth looked toward the white pillowcase she heard a click. Turning back toward the detective, she wondered if he'd pulled back the trigger on his handgun. Instead, she saw him holding the recorder where a small cassette tape was recording.

He paused, looking at her, anticipating an answer.

"I d-don't remember," she whimpered.

"Okay, your name, though?" he asked.

"M-m-my n-n-name, though," she repeated. Her eyes fixed again on the fluttering white pillowcase in the car just ahead of her. Dear Jesus, what was her father trying to tell her?

An earsplitting shriek accompanied by a horrific pounding erupted outside her car window. Yelping, Elizabeth cowered, covering her head with her hands.

"I said, time's up!" Her mother was beating on the passenger's side window with her fists. "Time's up!"

The Toy Room Officer appeared from nowhere, dwarfing her mother. He picked her up, swiveled around, and plunked her down away from the car. "You're wrong, Ma'am. Time's up when the detective says it's up. You best get yourself back up in that house unless you want an obstruction charge," he ordered.

Mom retreated toward the house, the Toy Room Officer now shadowing her.

Elizabeth wiped the tears from her face and wondered when she'd started crying.

The pillowcase had vanished, and disheartened, she realized she'd missed Dad's message.

Suddenly she was on the concrete porch, and Detective Sims was walking away from her. From afar she stared at her father's profile as he sat in the police car.

Please, Dad, look at me. Our secret's safe. I didn't tell anyone.

Dad's police car engine roared to life, and he never looked up.

Oh Jesus, he is leaving me here with Mom.

Forlorn, she entered her house, head down. She paused beside the Toy Room Officer. Reaching out, he placed his strong hand upon her shoulder. She looked up and their eyes met.

As she wiped more tears from her face she felt oddly safe beside him; she felt protected. She wanted to stand here forever. She knew her legs would not get tired.

The officer's hand left her shoulder. Footsteps approached, and someone cleared her throat.

Liz forced herself to look up and met her mother's raised eyebrows. Elizabeth slowly blinked once with both eyes.

Her mother smiled.

TWENTY-FOUR

Memory

The cabin on Banks Lake had been in Matt's family for at least twenty-five years. It was a popular, rustic, summer resort for the cousins and grandchildren. Elizabeth and Matt had spent most of Saturday swimming, fishing, and napping. They pitched their pup tent at dusk, since all the beds in the tiny cabin were already claimed by visiting cousins, nieces, and nephews. As evening descended, they roasted marshmallows over the campfire before retiring to their tent for the night.

Awakening to the smell of damp earth and a smoldering campfire, her eyelids fluttered at the morning sun dappling the side of the small turquoise pup tent. A loon called out, and the faint odor of dead fish wafted in through the screened mesh windows.

Dad's breath was suddenly upon her neck, and his smell overcame her. Gasping and now wide awake, she leaped, screaming, from their sleeping bag, lunging across the tent. On her knees, clutching her throat, her entire body trembling, seconds of memories washed over her.

"Lizzie and I will sleep in here tonight," he spoke, the green tent flashing before her, butter and salt mingling on her tongue. His calloused hand groped her breasts. She looked down, eyes gaping. No one's hands were there.

Her wild eyes darted left and right, then up and down.

He was not here.

He was not here.

Thank Jesus in heaven, he was not here.

The loons called to her again, sealing the crystal-clear memory.

There had been no headache when her father touched her that night in Canada.

Still trembling, she pulled her knees to her chest and closed her eyes.

"Liz?"

She jumped.

"Hey," Matt whispered. "Come here."

Forcing her limbs to move, she crawled atop the sleeping bag beside him. Allowing his arm to draw her in close to him, she slowed her breathing and prayed he wouldn't ask her any questions.

"Your heart's beating through your chest, you know." He raised himself up using his elbow. "Bad dream?" he asked.

Nodding, she closed her eyes and turned away from him.

"Think you can go back to sleep?" he asked.

"Yeah," she replied.

"Okay, let's get up in an hour and head for home."

* * *

After refueling at the first gas station in Greenville, she turned on the radio.

"Hold up," Matt said, turning it off. "What was your nightmare about?"

"It wasn't a nightmare." She hesitated. "You know I've been talking with Maureen about Dad and the back rubs? How he never knew what he was doing? Well, I think I know for sure now"—she paused—"that some of the time, he knew. At least once, anyway."

"No shit," Matt replied. "Of course he knew, and he knew *every* time."

She turned toward him, stunned. How could he be so certain?

"Sorry," he apologized.

She stayed silent.

"I mean it, I'm sorry," he repeated. "Keep going."

"It was when I woke up this morning. I remembered a time I was with Dad, and he didn't have a migraine. It was in a tent when my family went camping in Canada. That time, he knew," she said with a sense of resignation. "He knew what he was doing."

Matt reached over, grasping her hand.

"The headaches clouded the issue. He was in such pain—"

"No," Matt interrupted. "Sorry, but there was no headache or migraine or whatever he called it that day. He was never in pain.

When *you* have headaches, do you want me to touch you? Do you have conversations with people? No, you lie down and take an aspirin."

She looked at him, startled at how his words rang true, as if her hearing were tuned correctly for the first time.

"Liz, I gotta say if it weren't for you, I'd have beaten the shit out of that man a long time ago. So I don't mean to sound too happy, but I'm glad you see it. I'm relieved you see it. It's healthy to see him for who he is—a coward and a bully—a damned freak. So are you going to tell Maureen?" he asked.

She nodded.

"Good." They drove in silence for a minute or two.

"You know what?" he said. "This money we're paying for therapy? It's already the best investment we'll ever make."

TWENTY-FIVE

Auntie

Hearing another car start and looking out the window, she watched the Toy Room Officer ease into the detective's sedan. She felt a safety net falling away. Floundering in powerlessness, she closed her eyes and did not move.

"Your Uncle Jeff is here," her mother announced. "Thank God."

Opening her eyes, Elizabeth looked up to see a white car pulling into the drive. "I th-thought you hated Uncle Jeff."

"I do. But they have money," her mother replied. "Your dad needs a good lawyer."

Uncle Jeff and Aunt Sheila entered the house, and the adults huddled in the dining room. Elizabeth hid just inside the kitchen archway.

"…jail…Emma's lies…foster care…"

Elizabeth waited to hear her name, when she was leaving, and when she'd see her sisters.

"…lawyer…prison…fifteen years…"

Aunt Sheila poked her husband's arm with her elbow, clearing her throat. Her eyes darted toward Elizabeth and back.

Everyone stopped talking, and Elizabeth's mother strained a smile.

"Where's Ruthie, Liz?" Mom asked.

"In the s-s-sandbox with Todd."

"Could you go check on her? I need to talk with your aunt and uncle," she began. "Jeff, Liz is such a help. Thank God no one is taking her away from me. I don't know what I'd do."

The words sank to Elizabeth's stomach. She knew exactly what Mom was saying—she wasn't going anywhere.

"Becky?" offered Aunt Sheila. "Liz and I can check on the kids, so you two can talk."

Rubbing her forehead, Elizabeth's mother consented.

"Ready, Liz?" Aunt Sheila asked, walking toward the back door. "They have lots to discuss."

Now outside on the concrete porch, Aunt Sheila looked up at her niece.

"You're smiling," her aunt commented.

"Well, y-you're a little short," said Elizabeth. "You s-sort of stop where my neck starts."

"Perhaps." Aunt Sheila chuckled. "Or maybe you're just a giant girl."

Across the driveway, Todd sat motionless in the sandbox while William, Rachel, and Ruth played.

"They're doing well enough over there," Aunt Sheila surmised. "Let's go for a walk, shall we?" Without waiting for a reply, Aunt Sheila took her niece's hand in hers. The two walked the short distance to the driveway's end and made a right onto the gravel road.

Miniature white and lavender butterflies danced an erratic ballet alongside the gravel footpath that paralleled the river.

"Honey," began Aunt Sheila, taking a breath, hesitating. "We don't know each other well; actually, we don't know each other at all, do we?"

Elizabeth shook her head.

"We've met twice—maybe three times your whole life? Well, that's okay—because God made all of us, right?"

Aunt Sheila stopped. "Do you mind if I pray?" she asked, taking both of Elizabeth's hands in hers. "I know you're a Christian. I am, too. We don't go to the same church, but we pray to the same God, right?"

Closing her eyes, her aunt began without waiting for Elizabeth's reply. "Dear Jesus, thank you for Liz. We know she is Your child, and You love her so much. Put your arms around her, Jesus. Allow her to feel Your love. Help her to know I love her. Help her to trust me. It's so hard to know who to trust."

Elizabeth held her breath, her body aching for someone to trust. Unable to restrain her emotions any longer, she slumped forward, her forehead resting upon her aunt's shoulder. She sobbed.

Aunt Sheila's arms encircled her. "Jesus, give her courage to trust me just for today. In Your name. Amen."

Tears still flowing, Elizabeth wondered if she could trust her aunt.

"Here," she began, taking off her beige cotton sweater, "Let's sit on my sweater here on the side of the road. And you just go on and cry, babe," Aunt Sheila murmured. "You've got a lot to cry about. Here's a tissue, too" she offered, fumbling in her jeans pocket.

Elizabeth accepted the tissue as her aunt released her.

"Better?" Aunt Sheila asked after she'd blown her nose.

Elizabeth nodded. They both sat down, sharing the large sweater.

"Good. Now I need to ask you something," Aunt Sheila began. "And before you tell me anything, I gotta tell you that all I know about any of this is what I've watched on the *Phil Donahue Show*. But whatever you tell me, I won't tell anyone. I'm the best secret keeper that ever was."

Elizabeth looked up, raising her eyebrows at her aunt. "You won't tell anyone?"

"No one," she said.

"What about Uncle J-Jeff?"

"Not even Uncle Jeff," she promised.

"M-m-mom s-said th-th-that…" Her throat tensed with every breath, and she looked down and wrapped her arms around herself.

Tenderly lifting Elizabeth's chin from its lowered position, Aunt Sheila spoke. "Guess what," she quipped. "You stutter. And don't think I'm not used to it. Your Uncle Jeff stuttered when we first met. So you just take your time, because we've got all day. Now, take a deep breath and let it out."

While the tall, wild, black-eyed Susan's danced in the warm summer breeze, Elizabeth inhaled, then exhaled. Suddenly, it seemed as if time had found a safe place to stop.

"M-m-mom said th-that if I l-l-lied to the detective about the back rubs, I c-could be with Emma and Sarah in foster c-care. And if Emma and Sarah g-go with you and Uncle J-Jeff I get to go, t-too."

Aunt Sheila nodded her head. "Okay, anything else?"

"Mom said she's our g-g-guardian now, so she gets to say where w-we all go, and since Emma and S-Sarah are scared, and maybe g-getting r-r-raped—" Elizabeth's sobs overtook her again.

"Hold on, babe," Aunt Sheila replied. "First, your sisters may be scared, but scared never killed anyone before. And why would you think they're being raped?"

"M-mom said so," she sniffed.

"I don't know why she'd tell you that." She paused here for a long moment. "What else did she say?"

"If I t-t-told the truth about the back rubs, Dad w-w-would go to j-jail for fifteen years and b-be raped and sleep on a cement floor and eat br-bread and w-w…" Her voice trailed off into nothingness.

"Water?"

Elizabeth nodded, using the tissue again.

"Okay," her aunt soothed, placing a hand upon her niece's shoulder.

"M-mom said if I loved him, I would l-lie like she l-l-lied for her dad when it happened to her."

"She said it happened to her?" Aunt Sheila asked.

Elizabeth nodded again.

"Babe, can you tell me what *it* is? I mean, what your mother asked you to lie about?"

"The b-back rubs," she replied.

"Back rubs?" Aunt Sheila asked.

"Yeah. If I tell the t-t-truth about the b-back rubs, Dad will go to pr-prison."

Aunt Sheila surveyed her niece. "Liz, I don't have all the answers right now, but your mom is lying to you—maybe not about every-thing—but about some things. First, she has no say about Emma or Sarah, and she won't have any say about you in a matter of hours. From what I know so far, you'll all be in a foster home by the end of the day."

"B-but she said she's our g-guardian."

"She's not. She's not Emma's, Sarah's, or yours. All three of you are wards of the state. She doesn't know where your sisters are right now, and when that social worker finds a home for you, your mom won't know where you are, either. None of this is up to her." Aunt Sheila pursed her lips and shook her head. "She shouldn't have done this to you," she finished.

"You w-won't tell her, right?" Elizabeth sniffled, wondering if her aunt would confront her mother.

"What?" Aunt Sheila asked.

"Remember, how you promised not to tell?" Elizabeth whimpered.

Aunt Sheila placed her hands on Liz's shoulders. "You think I'm going to run and tell your mother everything you've just told me? Not a chance. You forget, babe, I've known her a long time. I know what she's like."

Elizabeth's tears slowed.

"I should slow down here, though. That might help you relax a little. Now here's my thinking: first, you know that your mother and Jeff aren't close. Let's be honest—they can't stand each other."

Elizabeth felt a smile interrupt the path of her tears.

"And I'm going to ask your permission for something. I know I said I wouldn't tell anyone what you told me, but I'd like to tell your Uncle Jeff a little of it—not all of it, just a little. Is that okay?"

"He'll tell her, won't he?" Elizabeth asked. "She's his sister."

"Liz, listen—the reason you and I don't know each other is because your mom and Jeff haven't talked for years. They don't get along. He came here—*we* came here—for you girls. Not for your mom. We found a babysitter and jumped in the car to get here as fast as we could. Plus, your Uncle Marty and Aunt Suzanne, remember Aunt Suzanne, your mom's sister? They're coming from Oklahoma City to help, too."

Elizabeth's eyes flickered. "You c-came for us g-girls?"

"We did. We came here for you and Emma and Sarah, not—"

Almost knocking her over, Elizabeth threw her arms around Aunt Sheila, a sob of relief escaping her.

Aunt Sheila gazed at her niece intently. "Trust me, dearie. You've got to trust someone, and you don't know it yet, but I'm your best bet. Let me and Uncle Jeff take care of your mother. Now, before we go back to the house, I need to ask you: do you want to go with me and your uncle to Colorado?" Aunt Sheila asked.

"With m-my sisters?" Elizabeth asked.

"I'll try, but I'm no miracle worker. And I'm not going to lie to you like your mom did to get you to do one thing or another. I know the home your sisters are in had room for two kids, and since you were on some kind of trip when the police got to your house, they just took your sisters. Even though you don't know us, if Jeff and I agree to be the foster home for you, is that better than you going to a stranger's house?"

Elizabeth trembled. "I d-don't want to go to a stranger's house without my sisters."

"Okay." Aunt Sheila paused. "Then here's my plan for now, and it may change because I'm flying by the seat of my pants. We'll go back to the house, and when we do, don't talk. Don't even look at your mom. Just get your stuff packed and wait upstairs for me to call you. We're leaving in ten minutes, and you're coming with us."

Elizabeth's heart swelled at the words *leaving*, *we*, and *us*.

"And the other kids? Can they come?" she whispered.

"I wish," Aunt Sheila replied shaking her head. "The officer and social worker I talked to said the charges involved you, Emma, and Sarah. Your mom still has say-so over the rest. If we take anyone else, Jeff and I could go to jail, and then we wouldn't be helping anybody."

Elizabeth's heart ached at the thought of leaving William, Rachel, and Ruth. At least Rachel and Todd were allies. But William and Ruth would have no one to protect them.

"We better go," her aunt said. "If we're taking you and maybe your sisters across state lines, there'll be calls to make and papers to sign."

Within minutes they were back at the house. Elizabeth stepped over a narrow crack on the concrete porch where a cluster of bright-yellow, tufted dandelions bobbed in the humid breeze. She wondered if she'd ever see her house again.

Aunt Sheila led the way inside the house, and Elizabeth found herself focusing on the black heels of her aunt's shoes. Her peripheral vision revealed her mother still talking to Uncle Jeff in the dining room.

Unobtrusively entering the bathroom, she scooped up the paper bag still holding her clothes from Cedar Point. Walking quietly to the stairwell, she ascended the stairs to her bedroom. She hadn't unpacked from her trip to Cedar Point—she hadn't had time. And since most everything she owned was in her paper bag, she was packed.

She was ready.

TWENTY-SIX

Knowing

Winter 1990, twenty-five years old

"I've been thinking about the lie Dad told about the pictures. If I knew of a time I gave him a b-back rub and he didn't have a headache, then I would know for sure he was lying about the sexual abuse. But he had a migraine every t-time."

"So your main question is whether or not he knew he was sexually abusing you when he had a migraine?"

"Yes," I confirm. "I see the pattern of lying, but since he had a migraine every time, I'll never know if he knew what he was doing or not."

"Knowing one way or the other, what would that mean for you?"

"That Dad's role in all of it is bigger. My view of Mom as all-powerful and all-knowing, and that she controlled everything from the back rubs to the barn, doesn't completely make sense to me now.

The abuse couldn't have happened without Dad and Mom working together. But I could never tell Dad that. I'm too much of a coward."

"You have to tell him what you decide or you're a coward?" she asks.

"If I c-c-can't stand up for the truth, then I must not believe it?" I realize I'm asking her the question.

"Are you asking if you don't tell him what you think, you're wrong for what you think?" she asks.

As I finish writing, I look up at Maureen, my pencil in midair. "Sorry, I'm thinking hard right now," I interject.

"I can tell," she replies genuinely.

"If I don't tell him what I think, it doesn't mean I don't believe what I think?" I clarify.

"Your truth is yours to do with as you choose," Maureen says. "Whether you tell him or not, your truth is the same."

"So I don't have to confront him if I think he's lying?"

"When you say 'confront,' what are you thinking?"

"Confront—like saying, 'you did this, and I know you did it.'"

"Liz, there are many ways of confronting. Some survivors have an imaginary conversation with their abuser; others write a letter, put it in a balloon, and set the balloon free. Some write a letter and burn it. Others write a letter and mail it. Some have a face-to-face confrontation. The lady in the newspaper took her perpetrator to court. The important part is knowing you get to choose if and how you confront.

"You don't need to put yourself in harm's way in order to know your truth. You're allowed to know your truth and keep yourself safe."

"I like that," I say. I sigh with relief.

"Choosing what to do with your knowledge is part of the process of taking control of your life. You're in charge of how you confront—no one else."

"And whether I decide to confront him or not doesn't make my belief about whether or not he's telling the truth any less true."

"That's right. Your thoughts are important because they are your thoughts—your truth. You don't need to confront your father, or anyone else, for that matter, to prove your thoughts are true."

Your thoughts are important because they are your truth. I write it in my notebook and underline it. I cross my last *t* and look up at her.

"That takes quite a load off," I say.

"Good," Maureen says, smiling, "because it's true."

TWENTY-SEVEN

The Letter

"Two today," I say, plopping down in my pink chair.

"Have I told you I've never had a client come so prepared, notebook and pen in hand?" Maureen says, smiling.

I smile back at her. I remind her I had to have a psychiatric evaluation last week for insurance purposes. This particular psychiatrist happened to be a man, and I had dreaded the upcoming appointment.

"It went okay, overall," I began. "At one point he asked why I felt the need to see my father. I answered him without thinking. I said, 'I must see him.' He asked, 'and why must you?'

"Now, that question made me think hard. After a few moments I said, 'Because he asks me to.'

"So get this: he says, 'You might consider not obeying your father all the time. It may benefit you to get some distance from him.'"

I pause, raising my eyebrows.

"If a *man* suggests I consider not seeing my father, and maybe this man is a father himself—why not think about *not* seeing my dad? So then *that* made me think about those ways of confronting you mentioned earlier. Remember?"

She nods.

"I chose the one about writing and wrote Dad a letter. I don't know what I'm going to do with it yet, burn it maybe. But I'm not worrying about that right now."

"Writing fits you," Maureen surmises.

"Will you read it?" I ask.

"I could," she replies. "Or you could."

I realize if I stutter on every word, Maureen won't mind. The meaning will be the same.

"Okay," I say, smoothing the two-page letter on top of my notebook.

I take a deep breath.

"*Dear Dad:*"

My voice quivers.

"Oh, crap, I'm gonna cry," I say, reaching for the tissues.

"Take your time," she says.

I begin again with another deep breath.

"*Dear Dad:*

"*I am writing to you to tell you that I will not be seeing you for a while. I do not want you to contact me by phone, mail, or in person.*

"When I was a child, I was supposed to be treated like a child. I was supposed to be treated like a daughter. I should have felt safe, secure, and happy. I should have been able to trust you.

"But when I was a child, I was not treated as a child. I was unhappy and scared. I wished you were dead and then felt guilty for wishing you dead. I felt unsafe. I was afraid and would pray to God that you would not have another headache."

The first tissue saturated, I reach for another one.

"I'm really fluent," I sniff admiringly, wiping my eyes and nose.

Maureen nods and I see her eyes are moist.

I clear my throat.

"A lot of the memories I have as a child are unhappy. I remember the time we went to Canada on our camping trip. You often speak of that trip and the fun we all had. You n-never mention the night you said, 'Lizzie and I will sleep in here tonight.' You did not have a headache then. When you slid your hand up my shirt, I was scared. I was little. I made myself go numb again.

"I did not like to touch your genitals. I would pull my little hand away, and you would return it. Every t-time I pulled my hand away, you would put your hand on top of mine and return it. I did not like you touching me. I did not like you kissing me.

"When I was a child, I did not have a voice. I was trapped in your house.

"When I was an adolescent, I had a voice, but I was t-t-terrified. I was trapped in fear.

"I am a young woman now. I have a voice. I am not afraid. My voice gives me the power to tell you that you do not have power over me anymore.

"I am unsure if I will ever be able to feel safe around you again. I am working at taking care of myself right now. I cannot be around someone who has betrayed my trust—the trust of a little girl. My voice tells you to leave me alone for now. Liz."

Closing my eyes, a soothing saltiness trickles over my lips.

"Powerful," Maureen whispers, also grabbing a tissue. "So powerful. Good for you, Liz."

She extends her hand to me, and as I reach out to grasp it, we both rise together and embrace.

TWENTY-EIGHT

William's Eyes

Steadying herself against the windowsill that held her belongings, her heart leaped to William, just thirteen years old. How could she leave him with Todd and her mother—two people she could not defend herself against?

"She's staying!" her mother shouted.

"No, Becky! She kept her end of the bargain, and you know what I mean. Now you need to keep yours," Aunt Sheila commanded.

Within the looming silence, Elizabeth felt her world revving up for a massive quake. An animal-like scream filled the air, and from her bedroom window Elizabeth saw Todd lurch from the sandbox and run for the house. Will, Rachel, and Ruth followed close behind.

"I said no!" screeched her mother. "I'm her mother!"

The door flew open, hitting the wall. "Mom?!" Todd's voice cracked.

"They're taking Liz!" their mother wailed.

"Sheila, go," said Uncle Jeff. "Get Liz in the car."

"No!" screamed her mother. "Damn you!"

"Stop it! Look at the rest of the kids!" Jeff yelled. "Swear to God, Becky, you try to make her stay, and we'll tell the cops what you did to her! She's gotta go anyway—you should be grateful she's coming with us!"

Appearing at the top of the stairs, Aunt Sheila touched her niece's arm. "Let's go," she directed.

"Y-you first," Elizabeth whispered, hugging her paper bag as she grabbed the hem of her aunt's shirt.

"She can go, but wait!" screamed Becky.

Elizabeth and her aunt froze in the stairwell.

"Let her say goodbye to the kids," pleaded her mother.

"Don't, Jeff," Aunt Sheila's voice entered the laundry room from the stairwell. "She's just trying to torture her."

Poking his head inside the stairwell, Uncle Jeff motioned with his hand for them to continue forward.

"Let's go," he ordered. "You first, Sheila. Then Liz, and then me."

"Keep moving, Liz," whispered Aunt Sheila. "Whatever you do, don't look back."

Elizabeth remembered Lot's wife.

The three had rushed the few steps to the door when a child's voice filled the room.

"Liz," William bleated.

Elizabeth slowed.

"Liz?" the same voice begged.

Elizabeth turned back, and as she did, the macabre family portrait gutted her.

Todd, glaring at Elizabeth, held a whimpering Ruthie. A forlorn, eleven-year-old Rachel leaned against her mother, her tears streaming down her face, against a backdrop of freckles.

And William stood to the right of all of them—alone. He ran both his hands through his hair, tears trickling down his face. His widening eyes darted about in desperation, crying out to her. *How can you leave me alone?* They seemed to say. *Sarah is gone, and you know how it is here.*

Overcome, Elizabeth dropped her paper bag to the floor, and as the thud broke the silence, Elizabeth's mother spoke.

"Your sister's leaving," she began. "Let's hug her and—"

Aunt Sheila reached down, grabbed the paper bag, and flung it toward her husband who caught the bag midair. Grabbing Elizabeth's hand, Sheila pulled her the rest of the way out the door. Running to the car door, she shoved her niece inside.

"Go, Jeff!" she ordered, sliding into the front seat. "Becky's coming!"

Elizabeth turned and looking out her back door window, gasping at the frenzied look upon her mother's face as she ran toward the car. Elizabeth slammed down the locks on her door.

Will came tearing out of the house racing toward the car. "Liz! Wait! Don't!" a guttural scream grabbed her heart through the car window.

The car began moving, and Elizabeth watched from the back window in horrific grief. Will continued his frantic race, arms pumping at his sides as he grew smaller and smaller.

A sob escaped her as she watched him slow to a jog and then fall to his knees. Her mother continued running after the car.

"Will," she whispered. "I'm so sorry, Will." Slumping down into the backseat, she held her wrenching stomach.

"Sheila?" Uncle Jeff sounded panicky. "Um, Becky's still running after us. She's running in the middle of the highway! Should we stop?" He began slowing.

"Are you kidding me? She wants you to stop. Keep going!" Aunt Sheila ordered.

Liz felt the car accelerate as she stayed hunkered down in the backseat, sobbing.

"Sheila?" Uncle Jeff's tone sounded hollow, unsure. "Look at 'Lizabeth. She's still crying Will's name. What do we do?"

"Calm down, Jeff. It's us or strangers, and we're more or less strangers to her. She's going to need some time. And slow down, now. You're doing eighty."

"Aunt Sheila?" Elizabeth whimpered as the car decelerated.

Aunt Sheila turned around, fixing her brown eyes upon her niece.

"I d-did the right thing?" Elizabeth gasped between sobs.

"Yes, you did the right thing," Aunt Sheila replied.

Elizabeth looked into Aunt Sheila's eyes—the eyes that came for her.

"And Will? P-please can we go back and get him? He's no trouble—" she begged.

"Liz, I know your heart is breaking, but believe me, Will is going to be okay. Lots of policemen are watching your mother now. She will have to be careful or risk losing him, too."

"If Mom ends up losing him, can he please come live with you, too?" Elizabeth begged.

"Absolutely. We'd take all of you kids if we could. And if the law lets us, Will is more than welcome to stay with us."

Elizabeth wiped her face with both hands. "Promise?"

"Have I lied to you yet?" Aunt Sheila asked.

Elizabeth shook her head back and forth once.

"Babe, I know it's hard. But no matter how hard it gets, I'll never lie to you."

Looking into her aunt's deep, brown eyes, she reminded herself her aunt had come for her. She could trust her. Just for today.

TWENTY-NINE

Pictures of Me

Earlier, Maureen asked me to bring in some childhood pictures. Today I brought in two: a 3x5 taken when I was in kindergarten and an 8x10 taken when I was nine years old.

She asks me to choose one, and I point to the 8x10.

"What do you notice?" she asks, peering at the picture and smiling.

"Well, this is my third-grade picture. The first thing I notice is how ugly I am, especially the hair. Look at it, all teased and puffed into that bouffant hairstyle I always hated. Mom insisted on fixing my hair that way. She'd do it about once a week and always the night before picture day. And on picture day, she must have used half a bottle of hairspray to keep it in place. And look at my

161

skin; it's so pale it's almost gray. My freckles are barely visible, like they've faded away."

"So you noticed the hair first," said Maureen. "And you hated it?"

"I *loathed* it. Mom would sit in a chair and have me sit on the floor right under her. It took a whole hour every time. She'd use her spit to moisten her fingers and then run her damp fingers through the little group of strands she'd combed before coiling it up. Then, she'd use those stupid bobby pins, two of them for each curl, and pin every curl so close to my scalp, I felt like a pincushion. Those stupid bobby pins poked me in the head all night long."

"What were you feeling during all of this?"

"Angry. And powerless. I hated how she'd lick her fingers with her bad-breath spit and wet my hair with it. I felt like I was going to explode. It was just one more reason to hate her."

"So you felt angry and powerless."

"Yeah, just another time I had no choice over my own body."

Maureen nods. "I notice the style seems old for a nine-year-old. This seems to fit the role your mother defined for you in your family."

Peering at this little girl, I shake my head. "I never knew looking at a little girl's picture could make me feel so sad."

"What part is sad?"

"She looks so tired, so spent. I *told* Mom how much I hated that hairstyle, and how the other kids laughed at me. She didn't care in the slightest. Couldn't she just let me wear my hair down and straight, so I didn't feel ugly? Shouldn't a little girl be allowed to feel pretty?"

Maureen nods.

"Now here in this one?" I hold up the 3x5 so it's facing Maureen, then lay it down in my lap. "This is my kindergarten picture. I'm much cuter here—no hair spray or pin curls—just a little ponytail in the back. My skin looks better, too, see? My cheeks are almost rosy and my freckles have pigment to them. I don't look all worn out. My eyes even sparkle a little."

"Any feelings about that picture?" Maureen asks.

"I look at her and feel happy, like, she's just a regular little girl." But Maureen's question raises a curtain upon the timeframe that separates these two pictures. My eyes travel back and forth between the two little girls looking at me from my lap—one cute, one ugly—and yet they are the same child. Or are they?

"Liz?" Maureen asks.

I point to the little girl in the 8x10 picture. "It's just, I was thinking about when I brought this picture home from school. I remember Dad saying, 'Maybe next time Mrs. Wellers should remind you to swallow your spit before they take your picture.' See that little pool of spit right there in the corner of my mouth? Mrs. Wellers was my third-grade teacher, and she had a student teacher that year, a man. I loved him. I mean, crush-like, little-girl love. I remember wondering about his headaches, if he had daughters, and if he had a favorite.

"You know something? I never knew for sure when the sexual abuse started—exactly I mean. But I always felt that I was about nine. And I gotta be close because in third grade you're nine. It must have been happening if I'd had those thoughts about that student teacher."

163

"So what you felt was right on," Maureen confirms.

"It was. And yet when I was interviewed after Dad was arrested, I couldn't seem to remember much of anything. I couldn't help Emma and Sarah prosecute Dad at all, even though I was the oldest, the so-called big-sister."

"Liz, as long as I've known you, the big-sister context has always included wishing you'd helped prosecute your father."

"It's true, and I'm not blaming anyone: not God, me, or anyone else. I was so little, around nine, when the abuse started, and by the time Dad was arrested I was sixteen. Somehow seven years of fear did something to me that made me less capable. By the time I was interviewed, I was beaten down to a stuttering, anxious, fearful, little girl."

"Do you remember much about that interview?" Maureen asks.

"Some, but not a lot." I shook my head back and forth. "It's one of those fuzzy, almost white slides in my life. I remember the detective was patient. He was trying to help me narrow down a specific time when I was with Dad in bed. And I remember *wanting* to tell the truth and ordering myself to *not* go into my wall during the interview. I know I said something about Halloween. And you know what else I remember? Smelling my mother."

Maureen raises her eyebrows.

"I know, weird, isn't it? Her perfume was nauseating."

"Smell is a powerful sense for many survivors."

I feel so normal when I'm with Maureen.

"So you remember bits and pieces of the interview. Have you told me before about Halloween? I don't remember that."

"I haven't thought about it until now," I said. "In our family, after your sixteenth birthday, you were too old to go trick-or-treating.

The Halloween I was fifteen, Dad had a headache, and it was my turn to go first. I knew it was my last year to go trick-or-treating, so I asked Mom if I could take two turns next time Dad had a headache and have Emma or Sarah take their turn this time. Mom said no, that it was more important that Emma and Sarah go trick-or-treating because they were younger.

"I was a gypsy that year." I smile at this part of the memory. "By the time the sun went down, I was wearing red lipstick, blue eye shadow, and black liquid eyeliner. I thought I was so beautiful. And then, he got a headache." My voice trails off. "But the day I was interviewed, I'm not sure what I said about Halloween. I remember saying the *word* Halloween—that's about it."

"So back when you were a teenager, and you weren't able to provide testimony, that's where this feeling that you never did anything comes from. And you wished you'd been more able to tell the truth, to be the big sister to Emma and Sarah? Does that fit?"

"It fits. And God knows, I wish it didn't fit. I wish I could go back now and whisper in that scared kid's ear—tell her what to say. But I can't. I just have to accept that I wasn't strong enough back then."

"I'm not sure this means you weren't strong, Liz. You had to be strong to survive your family. But if you *could* go back to that interview, what do you think you'd say?"

"First, I would name a specific time he sexually abused me. Then I'd tell Dad he knew what he was doing; I'd tell him to leave us all alone."

"So first, you'd name a time he abused you. Then you'd tell him he knew what he was doing. Then you'd tell him to leave you alone. I think you might have done something close to that. Here," Maureen murmurs, thumbing through her notes and handing me the letter I wrote to Dad. "Do you see the words I mean? It's near the Canada part."

Scanning my letter, I see it. "I remember the time we all went to Canada on our camping trip…You never mention the night you said, 'Lizzie and I will sleep in here tonight.' You did not have a headache then."

I smile ruefully. "I did write that, didn't I?"

"And you wanted to tell him to leave you and your sisters alone," she adds. "Here it is, near the end."

I scan the end of my letter: "I cannot be around someone who has betrayed my trust—the trust of a little girl. My voice tells you to leave me alone for now."

Another smile flits across my face. "It's late coming, but at least it's in there."

Looking down, I see the two little-girl pictures side by side in my lap.

I point to the younger of the two girls.

"Look how cute she is here," I said. And then I point to the 8x10 picture. "And then look at what they did to her here. She looks so tired, so alone. For so many years they did it to her—her whole childhood lost."

"Liz?" Maureen interjects. "Could you try that again, but use the word *me*, instead of *her*?"

"I can," I say, my chest tightening. "But I'd like to be strong enough to do it without crying."

"Liz, you are strong," Maureen reassures. "Talking through your tears is a sign of strength, not weakness." She leans back in her chair, as if we have all the time in the world.

"What I meant to say was"—I grab a tissue, press it against my closed eyes, and breathe in—"for so many years they did it to me. And I was so tired, and so alone." I take another cavernous breath as the tears flow down my face. "My whole childhood—lost."

THIRTY

Colorado

As she followed her aunt, uncle, and three younger cousins into their enormous, brick Colorado home with arching windows, Elizabeth could not comprehend such a small family living here. Speechless at the luxuries in front of her, she noticed each bedroom was carpeted, replete with matching curtains and bedspreads. There were wooden dressers with large oval mirrors and a bookshelf filled with books in each room.

Elizabeth, overwhelmed, was next led downstairs to *her* bedroom, and *her* bathroom. Her spacious bedroom had a queen-sized bed and a white down comforter, topped with sky-blue pillowcases with a white lace edging. A huge, oak, wooden dresser with a rectangular mirror sat across the room from the bed. In the corner, a Tiffany lamp sat upon a small, oak desk. The nightstand beside

168

her bed, also oak, boasted a clock radio, a smaller Tiffany lamp atop a white doily, and a box of tissues.

Across the hall, the cut-glass lighting in the bathroom filled the room with a warm soft, light. Entering the bathroom, she stepped upon the softest rug she had ever felt beneath her feet. Looking down, she saw it was made of what looked like sheepskin.

A gold towel bar held up two oversized, blue fluffy towels. Near the sink, there was another golden bar with a smaller blue towel and then a matching blue washcloth. A hook behind the door held up a white cotton robe. Walking toward the floral shower curtain, she drew it back and smiled.

"A shower," she whispered.

"Mmm, yes," Aunt Sheila murmured, looking around. "We'll bring shampoo and hair conditioner down after we eat. We weren't expecting company, but we're glad we have some."

Pausing, she cocked her head toward the thumping ceiling. "I hear the natives. Better get some food on the table."

The two walked up the steps and into the kitchen.

"Can I help?" asked Elizabeth approaching the kitchen counter.

"Hey, thanks," her aunt replied. "Silverware's right underneath you there."

Counting out the spoons, Elizabeth swallowed hard as she stopped at the number six. She looked up as her uncle entered the kitchen.

"Sheila," he said, "I've got a headache. I'm gonna go lie down for about twenty minutes."

Elizabeth froze.

Reaching above the microwave and opening a small cabinet door, Uncle Jeff fumbled for a moment with his right hand then withdrew a small red-and-white bottle. Elizabeth watched him pop the small round top off with his thumb. Turning the bottle on its side, he tapped out two round pills into his palm. Replacing the top with a firm click, he returned the bottle to the cabinet.

"I bet you're hungry, too," his wife replied. "Here's a little sandwich and some milk."

"Thanks," he said, throwing his head back and swallowing the tablets. He accepted a small plate with a ham sandwich and a glass of milk from Sheila.

Elizabeth watched him leave the kitchen, listening. His footsteps stopped near the family room.

"Carissa?"

"Yes, Daddy?" replied the eight-year-old.

"Turn the TV down, babe. I have a headache and can hear it from my room."

"Sure, Daddy," Carissa replied. As the volume lessened, Elizabeth heard her uncle's footsteps fading down the hall until a door closed.

Swaddled in relief and then confusion, she wondered if her uncle loved his daughters.

"Let's eat," said her aunt, and Elizabeth jumped.

"Sorry, didn't mean to startle you," she apologized.

Seated now with her aunt and three cousins, Elizabeth admired the ham-and-cheese sandwiches aligned on a bright white platter alongside glasses of milk, sliced apples, and bright orange carrots. About halfway through their meal, Uncle Jeff reentered the kitchen, and Elizabeth watched as he approached the table.

"Looks good," he announced, running his fingers through his hair. "Wait, though." Grinning, he went to the pantry, returning with a bag of potato chips. "These make it great!"

"Yes!" the children squealed.

"Headache gone?" Aunt Sheila asked, helping her daughters ration a reasonable portion of potato chips.

"All gone," he said. "And I *was* hungry. I think that sandwich helped as much as the aspirin."

Dinner was over, and Aunt Sheila showed Elizabeth how to load the dishwasher. After adding powdered soap to the receptacle and starting the dishwasher, her aunt sighed and then wiped her hands on the dish towel that hung near the stainless-steel kitchen sink.

"There. Dishes are done; kids are fed. We've been busy! Let's get everybody into bed. It's late."

Elizabeth chuckled at her aunt's interpretation of busy as she prepared to shower.

Downstairs after her shower, Liz slid between the bed sheets, realizing she had never slept alone before. Closing her eyes, she tried to pray but instead found herself yearning for Sarah's familiar arm dangling over her shoulder and the snuggling of her youngest sister, Ruth.

Aunt Sheila emerged from the hallway, knocking on the doorframe. "Nighttime will be hardest," she murmured. "I love you, babe," she said, stroking Elizabeth's forehead. "Can I pray with you?"

Elizabeth nodded, sliding over as her aunt sat on the edge of the bed.

"Father God," Aunt Sheila began as she grasped Elizabeth's hands. "We come to You, seeking Your strength, and let me just say—" her voice cracked, trailing off into a whisper.

Elizabeth opened her eyes to peer at her aunt's tear-stained face. "We need Your kind of strength for a burden this big. Strengthen Liz," she begged. "Strengthen Emma and Sarah, Todd, William, Rachel, and, um…"

"Ruth," Elizabeth whispered, giggling at her aunt's forgetfulness.

Aunt Sheila opened her eyes. "Yes, Ruth," she said sheepishly. "I knew that, I'm just tired. Anyway, He knew who I meant."

They both laughed. "And thank You, Lord, for that little bit of laughter. We needed that. Amen." Aunt Sheila gave her a quick hug. "Okay—try to get some sleep. It'll be better in the morning, I promise."

Alone in the new darkness, Liz replayed the past twenty-four hours. Her trip to and from Cedar Point was now a fog.

Her father, now in jail, might have a headache. She hoped the jail had some of her uncle's aspirin. Maybe then he wouldn't have headaches. She couldn't wait to get her hands on some aspirin herself. She had seen it work with her own eyes. It was magic.

Aunt Sheila reappeared, bringing a glass of water and a pink capsule.

"Here, this will help your stuffy nose. It might help you sleep, too."

Sitting up, Elizabeth took the medicine and placed the glass of water upon the nightstand.

"Don't think I'm insane," her aunt said, kneeling alongside the bed. "Do me a favor and try to think of one happy thought."

"Now?" Elizabeth asked.

"No, next Christmas," Aunt Sheila replied, rolling her eyes and smiling. "Yes, now, please."

Closing her eyes, Elizabeth thought for a moment, then opened them again, shrugging her shoulders.

"What about school? Any best friends or favorite teachers?"

"Mr. Morgan," popped out of Elizabeth's mouth.

"Favorite teacher?"

Elizabeth nodded.

"Good. Here's your job then," she ordered. "Think of Mr. Morgan for now. All the other stuff, you can think about tomorrow. But tonight, just think about him. Can you try that?"

Elizabeth nodded.

"Good," her aunt said. She tucked the sheet in beneath Elizabeth's chin and left the room again.

Lying between cool, crisp sheets, floating back to fifth grade, she sat at her brown desk. She was wearing her blue denim jumper. Mr. Morgan came to her like a feather on a billowy cloud. His brown eyes beckoned to her, and she smiled, feeling his warm hand upon her head.

Bending her neck to the right, her pillow became his comforting shoulder, and his strong, gentle arm hugged her bony frame. She was, after all, *his girl*, and he thought her brave and good.

She inhaled. *Ah, there it was—the scent of Old Spice.* A smile flickered across her lips, and she drifted off to sleep.

THIRTY-ONE

Big Sister

Winter 1991, twenty-six years old

I smile as I enter Maureen's ultra-warm office, take off my coat, and lay it across the back of my pink chair.

"Lots of snow, eh?" Maureen offers, yellow pad in hand.

I nod, settle into my chair, and a familiar sense of purpose presents itself. I know Maureen will ask me how I am—and she'll really want to know.

"Doin' okay today?" she asks.

"Yes, doing well I think," I reply, opening up my journal. "I've read the letter I wrote to Dad over and over. I'm wondering what might happen if I give it to him. I'm afraid if I give him the letter, I might regret it."

"Sometimes weighing the pros and cons is wise. What will be most important is making sure you are always safe."

"Let's start weighing then."

"What do you think will happen if you give him the letter?"

"It will kill my relationship with Dad, his relatives, and Todd."

"So the relationship with your dad, his relatives, and Todd will end. Anyone else?"

"Sarah loves me unconditionally, and Will does, too. They won't care either way. Emma's in New York and won't hear about it. And I don't think Rachel has a clue about the sexual abuse, so it won't affect her at all. Ruthie still lives with mom, so that's a nonissue. I could care less what Mom might think. It's just Dad, his relatives, and Todd."

"Let's look at your safety for a moment. From a safety perspective, what do you think your dad, his relatives, or Todd might do?"

"I'm not worried about Todd. I haven't spoken to any of Dad's relatives in years, so they'll likely just write me off, which would be fine with me. Now, Dad? I'm not sure." I pause. "When he divorced Mom, he stopped having anything to do with her. I hope that's how it ends with me, too. But it wouldn't be out of character for him to call my house and yell or swear at me."

"Okay, so imagine you're at home, alone. The phone rings, and you answer it. It's him, and he starts yelling and swearing at you."

I consider this.

"If I answer the phone and hear Dad's voice, I'll hang up. Plus, I could get caller ID or an answering machine to screen our calls. I can't imagine Dad just showing up at my house, because if he did, I'd call the police, and with his record, that would take care of him pretty quick. There are a lot of kids in our neighborhood."

"So, no matter how your dad or Todd responds, you're going to be physically safe?"

"I think so," I affirm.

"And you said the letter would 'kill' the relationship. How are you feeling about that?"

"I wonder if I'll feel guilty after giving him the letter because by giving it to him, I know it will end the relationship. So I'm purposely ending our relationship."

"You are familiar with guilt," Maureen says.

"I look at who was responsible for the sexual abuse, and now I feel I can see the whole picture in my head, logically I mean. I see it wasn't all Mom's fault. She was a key player and had her role in the abuse, but Dad's the perpetrator. He's the one who ended our relationship the first time he sexually abused me—and that's his shame, not mine."

"So on a cognitive level—in your head, as you said earlier—you see your father as responsible for the abuse and your mother as playing a part in it?"

"Yes. Mom could've been a heroine and saved us three girls from him, but she didn't. I think I was so hurt by that, for many years I placed all the blame on her. And I was so afraid of Dad, I couldn't consider he was responsible. I've punched Mom before; I knew I could overpower her. I've never punched Dad because I knew he could always overpower me."

"You had a lot to be afraid of," Maureen confirms.

"I did, and remember when we talked about me lying to stay away from him? To keep myself safe? Every conversation I have with him is pretty much a lie, because I feel I have permission to keep myself safe so I make up some reason not to see him. So over the past year, I think I've seen Dad once. I don't think that's much of a relationship. I mean, by giving him the letter, I won't see him at all…so I'm going from one time a year to zero." I shrug.

"So not seeing your dad at all if you give him the letter won't be much different from how much you're seeing him now?"

"Exactly."

"And you're comfortable with that?"

"I think so," I say. "And I think I'll feel less anxious, because I won't be worrying about seeing him again."

"Liz, what made you consider giving him the letter?"

"All the lying. I shouldn't have to lie to keep myself safe. I don't think God holds it against me that I've lied to keep away from dad, but that doesn't mean I have to live that way. I think God must be very fond of me, because God hates lying but I know He understands why I lie and loves me the same. On a basic level, I know in my heart He wants me to be safe. But lying is just one coping skill among many, and if I want to see myself as an honest person, I think I need to find a different way to stay safe. Maybe giving him the letter is an option; I don't know for sure yet. It's a caveat, don't you think? In order to consider giving Dad the letter so I can feel safe, here we are discussing whether or not by giving him the letter I can remain safe."

"So I notice two things here: One, it sounds like you want a more permanent sense of feeling safe, where you don't have to keep lying to stay safe?"

"Yes, a permanent sense of safety is what I'm going for. I'm tired of worrying about when I have to see Dad next."

"That takes a lot of energy," Maureen adds.

"It does, and it's a slow, constant drain."

Maureen nods.

"Something else is, by giving him the letter, I'm standing up to him. I'm behaving like the big sister."

"That's always been important to you," Maureen replies.

"It has. I'm okay now with how it was back then, how I couldn't say my name, much less give a statement. I'm focusing on the now. I mean, I can say my name *now*. And *now* I can write him a truthful letter. I may even end up giving him the letter. I'm pushing forward, not staying stuck in the past."

"You have come a long way, Liz."

"I have. And when I showed my letter to Sarah, you know what? She's going to write Dad a letter, too. I didn't ask her to write one. She just decided to do it after she read mine. That meant a lot to me. My little sister wants to do what I did. After all these years, I *feel* like the big sister."

Then I remember. "What else did you notice?"

"Oh, yes, the big-sister issue first…" She looked down at her notes. "And then, do you think you view God differently now than you have in the past?"

"Yes, my view of God has changed. He's not so scary and eager to send me to hell for lying to stay safe. Since I don't have a safe father here on earth, I think I've substituted the heavenly Father for my dad. It's safer trusting God than Dad, that's for sure."

"I like that expression you used about God being fond of you," Maureen replies.

"I like it, too," I say. "I like it a lot."

THIRTY-TWO

Interview

Her refuge came with a price tag named Will, Rachel, and Ruthie. And had she not abandoned her brother and sisters in Michigan, she could've forsaken her old life for the safety and comforts of her new one.

The imminent danger, the back rubs, were a thing of the past. Now her distress emanated from a different source—the encroaching trial date. Darkened circles beneath her eyes revealed an almost constant state of sleeplessness. Blackened cold sores crusted over her lips, cracking and bleeding as she used a straw to drink her food. She stuttered on nearly every word. The grimacing and straining required for each utterance proved too much, and in her despair she grew increasingly mute.

179

She knew she had to make a choice—she could continue to lie as her mother had directed, or she could tell the truth.

She knew the difference between the truth and a lie.

The truth would destroy her father and cause him to hate her. She would never be his favorite again. And yet, the truth would save her from certain hellfire.

The lie would save her father from prison, preserve the only love she'd ever known, and allow her to go home on behalf of William, Rachel, and Ruthie. But lying would likewise guarantee her place in eternal hellfire.

Her religious upbringing ensured a thorough understanding of the everlasting horrors of hell, and this proved the critical factor. She chose to think long-term; she chose to tell the truth.

She confided her decision to her aunt, who promised to stay with her when she gave her statement. The next day they were on their way to Michigan to see the prosecuting attorney.

Arriving at the dark-red brick courthouse that also served as the county jail, Elizabeth sat for a moment in the car and did not unbuckle her seat belt.

"I won't see him? You promise?" she asked from the backseat.

"He's on a work-release program, babe. He'll be at work," Aunt Sheila assured.

"Or Mom?" she asked.

"She's not supposed to know we're here, but if she is, you don't have to talk with her. We won't leave your side," Uncle Jeff promised.

Uncle Jeff led the way, and the three entered the building. They found the secretary's cubicle at the forefront of a well-lit corridor illuminating shiny linoleum floors. Lining the corridor walls were four doors, spaced evenly apart. Outside each door was a lone black chair, and in the farthest chair, a woman wearing black slacks sat, her head lowered.

"We're here to see the prosecuting attorney?" Uncle Jeff said to the secretary. The secretary picked up the phone, dialed, and said she would hold.

A police officer emerged from the first hallway door on the right, escorting a handcuffed, ankle-chained man in an orange jumpsuit toward the end of the corridor. Recognizing the back of her father's head, Elizabeth slipped behind her aunt.

Her father and the police officer approached the woman at the end of the corridor. The woman rose from her chair, and the pear-shaped frame of her mother was unmistakable. Both adults and the policeman entered the doorway to the left, closing the door behind them.

"The prosecuting attorney is here and wrapping up a meeting," replied the secretary hanging up the telephone. The telephone began ringing. "He'll be here soon. Excuse me, please. I need to answer this."

As she took the next call, a thin man wearing a dark suit and tie exited the same room the officer and her parents had just entered. He carried a black briefcase. His shoes clicked across the linoleum floor as he approached the cubicle. He exchanged handshakes with Uncle Jeff and Aunt Sheila and smiled at Elizabeth. She wondered if she should trust a man who had just been talking with her parents behind closed doors.

He beckoned them to follow him down the corridor, and Elizabeth balked. Where was he taking them? She had not agreed to this.

Aunt Sheila grasped Elizabeth's hand. "It's okay. You don't have to see your parents. Trust me. We'll do the interview and then head right back to Colorado, okay?"

"Okay," Elizabeth whispered.

They walked a few feet down the corridor and then entered the first room on the right.

Elizabeth held onto Aunt Sheila's hand and suddenly wished she hadn't come.

They entered the room where a too large, rectangular table hosted just two people. Elizabeth's pulse quickened as she recognized one face: Detective Sims. By now he knew she had lied to him the first time.

"First, let me say thank you for bringing Elizabeth here. I know you've come a long way," began the prosecuting attorney as he sat down in a chair. He placed his briefcase on top of the table. "Have you met everyone here?" he asked.

"No," Uncle Jeff replied.

"Detective Sims," said the prosecuting attorney, extending his hand toward the detective. Detective Sims stood then leaned over the table and shook Uncle Jeff's and Aunt Sheila's hands.

"And Mara Richardson, from Social Services." Mara Richardson also stood and shook Uncle Jeff's and Aunt Sheila's hands.

"Okay, now that we're all acquainted," continued the prosecuting attorney, "we can get started. Jeff and Sheila? If you'll step out and wait for us in the lobby near the secretary's desk, we'll try to make this as painless as possible. We know it's a stressful time for everyone."

Elizabeth jumped.

"Can I stay?" Aunt Sheila asked. "I promised I'd stay with her."

"I'm sorry, but we have to follow procedure to make sure her statement is admissible in court," explained the prosecuting attorney. "I'll call for you both as soon as we're finished. Okay?"

Angry tears filled Elizabeth's eyes. She refused to let go of Aunt Sheila's hand as the tears began trickling down her face. She heard footsteps outside the door and turned toward it, but no one entered.

Sheila held up her index finger in the silent room. "One minute with her? I'll talk so you all can hear me," she said.

The prosecuting attorney nodded, granting permission.

Turning toward her niece, she spoke. "Liz, don't be mad at them, be mad at me. I've never done this before, remember? I told you that the first day at your house."

Elizabeth felt her heart breaking.

"Besides, they're right. This needs to come from you. Now"—she reached in her purse and pulled out a small packet of tissues, pressing them into her niece's hand—"we'll be right outside in the—"

She could smell her mother's perfume.

"—M-mom's here," she said to her aunt.

"Yes," her aunt replied, "but she's in a separate room way down the hall."

Liz shook her head. "N-no. I smell her," her voice strained.

An awkward silence followed, then Aunt Sheila cleared her throat. "You can do this," she said, grasping Elizabeth's shoulders. "We'll be waiting for you right out there in the lobby."

Liz turned toward the still-closed door, narrowing her eyes. Didn't they know her mother was here? Couldn't they smell her? What was wrong with these people?

Or maybe, could it be? Her heart began beating so hard she placed her right hand over her breast. Perhaps this was how they'd planned it all along! What if, as her aunt and uncle left, her mother was supposed to enter?

Aunt Sheila and Uncle Jeff opened the door to leave, and Elizabeth's nostrils were contaminated with the stench of her mother's perfume. Her chest tightening she prepared to run should her mother take one step over the threshold.

But her mother was not in the doorway. Elizabeth, now perplexed, froze in place.

Detective Sims invited her to take a seat. Turning around, she paused and examined his face. He did not appear angry. She sat in the chair across the table from him and the social worker, adjacent to the prosecuting attorney.

Detective Sims retrieved a small black tape recorder from his suit coat. Pressing the black record button, he identified himself, the prosecuting attorney, the social worker, and then Elizabeth.

"Do you go by Elizabeth?"

"L-L-Liz," she stammered.

"Okay, Liz."

A familiar cough—her mother's cough—echoed from the hallway. Elizabeth turned around, held her breath, and waited for the door to open.

"Liz?" Detective Sims asked.

She turned back toward Detective Sims's voice, and the walls behind him called to her. She tried not to blink. She must hear the questions in order to tell the truth. An image of hell flashed through her mind.

"Mom said I should lie about the b-back rubs, like she did."

Turning around she saw there was no keyhole in the doorknob. The door couldn't be locked. Was there nothing to stop her mother from coming in?

"Liz? Do you remember a specific time…?"

Elizabeth turned back toward Detective Sims and cleared her throat.

"Halloween," she began.

Outside the door, chair legs scraped the linoleum floor, and Elizabeth winced. She blinked, and the humming began. Waving her hand in front of her face, she attempted to diffuse the stench of her mother's perfume.

"Are you too warm?" asked Mrs. Richardson.

"N-no," Elizabeth replied. Words swirled around her; sometimes the words came from Detective Sims, sometimes from Elizabeth's own mouth. Awhile later, Mrs. Richardson glanced toward Detective Sims and the prosecuting attorney. With a subtle nod from both, she reached for the telephone on the table and pressed some numbers.

Moments later, Aunt Sheila and Uncle Jeff reentered the room. Elizabeth rose from her chair and the tissue package dropped to the floor.

"You did it," Aunt Sheila affirmed, wiping the tears from Liz's face with her bare hand. Uncle Jeff took Elizabeth's right hand and squeezed it.

"Straight to the car," Aunt Sheila whispered. "Your mom's right outside the door. Don't look at her." Elizabeth clung to Uncle Jeff's hand as Aunt Sheila covered her from behind. Eyes downcast, she exited the room, following the heels of Uncle Jeff's leather brown shoes. In her peripheral vision, Elizabeth saw her mother's menacing black slacks seated in the chair just outside her door.

"Mrs. Luther, please come in," said the prosecuting attorney. And then his voice was cut off as the door closed behind her mother.

Outside in the parking lot, Elizabeth turned and looked behind her.

"She won't follow us. It's her turn to be interviewed," Aunt Sheila assured.

"Her turn?" Elizabeth asked.

"Yes. Let's just say she has some explaining to do. Did you tell them your mom asked you to lie the first time you spoke to Detective Sims?"

Elizabeth closed her eyes. She couldn't remember what she'd said. "I think so. I d-don't know."

"I'm sure you did fine," Aunt Sheila replied, patting Elizabeth's back.

"I hope so," Elizabeth said. "Because I d-don't think I c-could do it again."

THIRTY-THREE

Deliverance

"We gave Dad the letter," I said, before I was seated.

"We, as in you and Matt?"

"Yes, we made a plan," I continued, situating myself in my pink chair. "We were scheduled to go to Dad's for Christmas, so we thought we'd go and at the end of the visit, I'd offer to warm up the car, I'd leave, and Matt would give Dad the letter. If I changed my mind, I wouldn't offer to warm up the car, and Matt would hold on to the letter."

"What would've had to happen to cause you to change your mind?"

"Well, if Dad was somehow different, or maybe if he'd apologized, or some miracle like that. Or maybe I just wanted to give myself room to chicken out."

187

"So he wasn't different; there was no miracle; and you didn't chicken out?" Maureen asks.

I smile. "Right. Nothing had changed. In fact, while we were there, I told Dad I'd talked with Emma and thought I'd offended her. I said I needed to call her back and apologize. He laughed and said, 'Just drop it. If you don't think about something long enough, you forget about it, like water off a duck's back.' I've heard him use this expression before, but this time I realized it's a precept for him. It's how he lives his life.

"So after dinner and exchanging gifts, it was time to go. I said, 'Guess I'll go warm up the car' and kissed my dad on the cheek, knowing it would be the last time I'd ever kiss him. I was surprised at how serene I felt. The kiss wasn't poignant at all. It was"—I hesitate, trying to find the precise word—"perfunctory."

"Why do you think you were feeling so calm?"

"I knew he couldn't hurt me anymore. I was feeling brave—not so brave I could give him the letter myself, but brave enough to follow through. On my way out to the car, I heard Matt say, 'Del, here's a letter. Liz wrote it, but consider it from both of us. By the way, not *all* water runs off a duck's back.'"

"What happened next?" Maureen asks.

"After Matt got in the car, I told him he better hit the gas because he was now my partner in crime, so to speak. He put the car in drive and said, 'I think you're confused. That'd be your parents, not us.'"

Maureen smiles.

"I know, I like him too," I reply with a smile. "On the way home he asked if I'd caught the 'water off a duck's back,' statement. I told him I had. Then Matt said I'd been acting different around Dad this past year, not so jittery. And he said Dad had noticed it, too. I asked him why he thought this, and he asked me to compare last year's Christmas gift from Dad to this year's. That's when I got what he was saying."

"What did he get you last year?" Maureen asks.

"He got me a red-and-black lace negligee."

Maureen raises her eyebrows.

"Yes, that's what I think now, too, but just a year ago I felt so ashamed, like it was somehow my fault."

"And this year?" she asks.

I smile at her mischievously. "He got me an answering machine."

THIRTY-FOUR

Old Times

Fall 1981, sixteen years old

It was their first court-approved visit. Emma and Sarah, now living in Oklahoma with their Uncle Marty and Aunt Suzanne, arrived in Colorado, and the three girls clamored around one another, giggling and hugging.

After dinner, they went upstairs to the master bedroom and lay upon the king sized bed. Lying on their stomachs upon Aunt Sheila's bed, Elizabeth, Emma, and Sarah gathered, their three heads forming a triangle.

"What do you like most?" Emma asked.

"No b-back rubs and no barn," Elizabeth replied.

Crossing her wrists, Sarah rested her chin on the back of her hands. "Do you miss Mom?" she asked Elizabeth.

Elizabeth shook her head no.

"We don't miss Dad, either," Emma said.

"Liz, did he tell you it was a secret?" Sarah asked.

Astonished, Elizabeth stared at her younger sister. How did she know this?

"And that other people in the church did it, too?"

"No duh," Emma replied, rolling her eyes. "Like Randy and Lois?" Elizabeth froze. Her stomach turned. Emma and Sarah both knew? These were *her* secrets! Her father said that she was his favorite. Had the two somehow overheard Dad talking to her?

"And did he say you were his favorite? Or that if he didn't have you, he would die?" asked Emma.

Elizabeth felt as if she'd been punched in the stomach.

"Oh, and that he loved you the best?" Sarah interjected.

"Oh yeah, forgot about that one," Emma snorted.

Elizabeth's mind produced the only explanation to these revelations: her father had told Emma and Sarah these things to avoid hurting their feelings. After all, she herself was his favorite. He had told her so himself.

"Did he have you start out rubbing his neck and chest?" Sarah shuddered and stuck out her tongue. "He's so hairy."

Elizabeth's stomach twisted. He *was* hairy.

"Liz, did you hear Mom's filing for divorce?" Sarah asked.

"Hold up," interrupted Emma. "*Supposedly* filing—she's doing it so she gets to call us," said Emma. "It's just a trick to get us all home again."

"I heard we don't have to talk to her though," Sarah interjected. "Liz, did you hear that?"

Elizabeth shook her head no. Her heart was still reeling from her sisters' revelations. She knew nothing about a divorce or telephone calls. After the prosecuting attorney learned her mother had asked her to lie, her mother hadn't been able to contact her at all…and that's how Elizabeth liked it.

"Guess if there's a trial, we all have to go back to Michigan to testify. Do you get the plea bargain thing?" Emma asked.

Elizabeth shook her head in confusion, wondering what else she didn't know.

"Us neither," Sarah began. "It's something like Dad can say he did it with me and not Em, or with Em and not me, but he doesn't have to admit to both."

Perplexed, Elizabeth wondered why her name wasn't included in this 'bargain.' Was it because she didn't do a good job when she went to Michigan to speak with the prosecuting attorney? Had she stuttered too much?

"You think Mom will divorce Dad? I don't," Emma revealed.

"I do," Sarah replied. "Aunt Suzanne said if Mom wants us to come home, she has to."

"I'll believe it when I see it," Emma scoffed. "She'll say she's divorcing him, sure, but she won't go through with it. I'm telling you, she's just doing it to get us all home."

"Em could be right," Elizabeth offered. "One thing for sure is, you can never trust Mom."

After her sisters returned to Oklahoma with Aunt Suzanne and Uncle Marty, Elizabeth approached Aunt Sheila about the plea bargain.

"It's when you get to admit to some of the wrongdoing, but you don't have to admit to all of it," she explained. "Usually you get a lighter punishment."

"So Dad could admit to Emma or Sarah but not b-both?" Elizabeth asked.

"Yes," Aunt Sheila confirmed.

"Will he admit to me?" Elizabeth asked.

"Babe, I don't think so, just Emma or Sarah."

"It's because I d-didn't do g-good in Michigan, isn't it? Did I st-stutter too much? Do they think I'm lying?"

"Liz, no one thinks you're lying. You did your best, babe, and that's what matters," she soothed.

"So Dad c-can l-lie by admitting to Sarah, and it will help him get a lighter punishment if he lies?"

Aunt Sheila nodded.

"How can lying to a judge be okay?" Elizabeth pressed, her face reddening.

Aunt Sheila shrugged her shoulders. "It isn't okay. I mean, it shouldn't be okay."

"And the girls said something about Mom calling. Is Mom allowed to c-call me?" Elizabeth asked, her stomach tightening.

"I didn't want to tell you until I knew for sure." Her Aunt sighed. "But yes. We got word your mom filed for divorce, so she'll be allowed to call you girls."

"Do I *have* to t-t-talk to her?"

"Yes, and I tried to make it so you didn't have to, but this new social worker thinks your uncle and I have a grudge against your mom."

"What?!" Elizabeth exclaimed. "Didn't you tell her Mom asked me to lie about the back rubs and the turns?"

"I did," said Aunt Sheila softly. "The thing is, Liz, your mom denied asking you to lie. She said she didn't see you until a detective asked to interview you. Since no one saw your mom talking with you prior to your interview, it's her word against yours."

"But she's the liar here," Elizabeth continued. "Todd knows it. He's the one who told me to meet her in the bathroom."

"Honey, Todd isn't going to come forward with that information."

"So I told the truth this time, and they don't believe me?"

"The detective believes you; so does the prosecuting attorney. But they can't *prove* your mom asked you to lie, because no one saw her talking to you."

"Wait! What about Mom setting up all the shifts for the back rubs? Doesn't that prove Mom shouldn't be allowed to call me?"

Sheila rounded the kitchen counter and drew closer to her niece. "Your mom said you *girls* made up the 'turns' idea with your father, like it was between you kids and your dad. She said she never heard of it."

"What about Aunt Suzanne?" Elizabeth asked incredulous. "Did she talk to Aunt Suzanne? If she did, she'd see all of us girls are saying the same thing, and Mom's the one who's lying!"

Aunt Sheila sighed again. "Yes, and Suzanne got the same impression—that the social worker thinks all of us are against your mom. We have to remember, your mom fooled everyone in your church for years. It's probably pretty easy for her to trick one social worker."

"This w-worker's never even talked to me," Elizabeth spat.

"I know, babe. I think she's overworked."

"Or stupid," retorted Elizabeth, angry tears streaking her face.

"Or stupid," her aunt agreed.

THIRTY-FIVE

Attorney

"I was wondering," I begin. "Do you remember the name of the attorney who represented that lady in Marshall—the woman who sued her dad for sexually abusing her?"

"I remember the article but not the attorney's name. I'll see what I can find out, though," Maureen replies, getting up and jotting down a note on a Post-it.

"I'd like to talk with that attorney or maybe the lady she represented. I'm thinking about taking Dad to court for my own sense of justice. I mean, I never participated in the first trial. I wasn't involved in the plea bargain part of his jail sentence. I'd sure like to send Dad my own message."

"What kind of message?"

"That six months in jail for molesting three little girls isn't close to what I would consider justice."

"So you're seeking justice?"

"I suppose I am. And whether or not I end up having a case is pretty much immaterial to me. I feel called to do this—it feels right to me." I pause for just a moment. "But there are times I second-guess myself and slip back into this guilty, scary whirlpool."

"Liz, how old were you when you were removed from your home?"

"Sixteen," I reply.

"How long have you been in therapy?"

"Three years."

"So for sixteen years, you were trained to feel guilty and lived in fear. And for three years, you have done an enormous amount of work to heal. What do you know that can combat that guilty, scary whirlpool?"

"That it's not my fault, none of it. I remember when I first came to you, I felt so afraid and so guilty all the time. Identifying the back rubs for what they were—sexual abuse—helped me see it wasn't my fault."

"So naming it—calling it what it was—that helped you see you weren't the problem."

"Yes. I never realized that what you call something matters. And I never considered before that it wasn't my fault. But adults are in charge, kids are not."

"Yes, children are never at fault for sexual abuse," Maureen confirms.

"And the fact that I was sixteen had a hold on me, too. I felt I should have been the one to stop it, for me and my sisters. Or at least I should have been old enough to testify after the abuse came out. But now I see that by enduring the sexual abuse until I was sixteen, I was weakened. I wasn't strong enough to testify back then, because I'd endured the abuse for a long time."

"Liz," Maureen interjects, "I see you as being strong then, but not knowing much about your strength. You survived *years* of abuse. You wouldn't have been able to survive had you been, as you say, weak."

I let her words sink in. "I must have had some strength back then, otherwise I wouldn't have been able to breathe in and breathe out long enough to survive my parents. But I see a different kind of strength in me now, or maybe it's just a louder kind of strength. I'm strong enough to know the truth, and strong enough to write it. I'm strong enough to say it out loud, too."

"You are strong, Liz. You've always been strong."

A contented, tired sigh escapes me.

"I feel like it's time to stand up. It feels good to *be able* to stand up. Guess I'll find out what standing up to Dad looks like."

THIRTY-SIX

Decision

The first phone call from her mother was the template for all subsequent calls. Like a seasoned telemarketer, Rebecca advertised her new and improved family, struggling to live without the eldest daughter.

"You know, your father loves you so much, that's why he plea-bargained, so you wouldn't have to testify with your stuttering and all."

A despondent Elizabeth did not reply. She knew it would do her no good. The courts and social worker were all on her mother's side. The truth did not matter.

"And I've filed for divorce. You never have to see your father again."

More silence.

"And I'm seeing a counselor." Her mother cleared her throat. "Maybe after you're home, we could get off food stamps. With your dad in jail, there's no money, but if you were here, you could watch the kids while I worked. Todd's in the army now, so he can't help me."

Next, her brother and sisters spoke with her for about one minute, each parroting their mother's whispered coaching.

Her mother would then get back on the phone and ask Elizabeth if she was ready to come home.

"No," Elizabeth would reply. "Bye." Hanging up the phone, she'd race to the bathroom and vomit. It hurt to throw up. Canker sores still covered the outside of her lips and most of them were blackened and cracking, bleeding as she retched over the toilet.

At least, she considered, her reprieve had begun anew, and she wouldn't have to worry about the phone ringing for six more days.

But six days passed, and as 4:30 p.m. approached, Elizabeth took her place beside the telephone. Her mother was never late, proving herself a "fit and responsible" parent by calling each week at precisely 4:30 p.m.

The dreaded ringing began.

"I need to give William the phone for a sec," her mother said, just as Elizabeth answered. "Ruth's throwing up. I think she's got the flu. I'll be back in a jiffy."

And William was speaking. "Hey," he said.

"Hey," she replied.

"I'm supposed to tell you about the new place," he began. "It's got two showers, and we all get our own room. What, Mom?" he shouted.

Elizabeth paused. "How'd Mom get the money for such a nice place?"

"She sold off everything—the old house, the cottage on Diamond Lake and the forty acres of woods. Plus, she gets Dad's paycheck every week. She said where he's staying, he doesn't have to pay any rent. She's not making any payments either. This guy keeps coming by, because she hasn't made a house payment since we moved in." Will cleared his throat. "I'm supposed to tell you we're not going to church anymore." He chuckled. "That's one good thing that's happened since you left.

"Liz?" he whispered.

"Yeah?" she whispered back.

"Mom's worse," he whispered. "She's hitting us every day. She's drunk most of the time."

Elizabeth was silent.

"You hear me?" he pled.

"I hear you," she replied, panicking.

He cleared his throat. "Yeah, a fireplace, too." William proffered, "Mom's back—gotta go. Bye."

A hasty good-bye ensued as her mother's voice bit through the telephone lines. "Liz, what'd you say to make William cry?"

"Nothing," Elizabeth replied, "I didn't know he was crying."

"Listen up," she retorted, "I've divorced your father, and if that doesn't prove I love you, I don't know what will. You know my faith forbids divorce, but I did it for you. And if I've learned anything in counseling, it's this: it's my job is to take care of my kids. Your little game here, making us beg you to come home, is cruel." She paused. "So I guess I have to make a decision here. When I call next week, you're going to have to choose—rich relatives or us. I won't allow you to torture the younger kids like this."

A stilted silence hung in the air.

"Elizabeth, are you there?"

"Yes," Elizabeth refrained from asking her mother if daily alcohol use and smacking her kids around was part of *taking care of the kids*.

More silence.

"I love you," her mother said.

A silent Elizabeth removed the telephone from her ear, replaced the receiver, went to the bathroom, and threw up.

That night as she tried to sleep, William's desperation became her own.

She couldn't tell Auntie about William's comment. Her aunt would tell the social worker; the social worker would interview William or share the information with their mother. And then he would get it.

This was between her and William—no one else.

The next morning, enduring school in an anxious haze, she requested a restroom pass from her first hour-teacher. Standing at the mirror, she met a hollow, desperate reflection. Dark circles lived beneath her eyes and drew further attention to her blackened cold sores. Closing her eyes she wondered where William was right now. A knife twisted inside her as she realized she had a safe place to go home to every day; he did not.

Elizabeth had been praying for a miracle. Maybe God would strike her mother dead or otherwise render her "away." Today, she realized there would be no miracle. Reality, she knew, was void of miracles.

Rather than return to class, she went to the office and requested permission to call her aunt. As the first word left her mouth, however, Liz began crying and no matter how hard she tried, she could not stop.

Soon after, the school counselor, a tall, beautiful Asian woman with raven hair and creamy skin introduced herself, inviting Elizabeth into her office. Patting Elizabeth on the shoulder and motioning for her to sit in the high-backed chair, she passed Elizabeth a box of tissues. Next, the counselor closed the door, took a seat at her desk, and opened a manila file folder.

"You're living with your aunt and uncle? Is that going okay?" she asked.

Elizabeth nodded.

"And school? Is school going okay?"

Elizabeth shook her head no.

"Can you tell me why?" she probed.

Elizabeth wept. Overcome, she revealed her dilemma. Her father was in jail, her brother was afraid, and her mother was worse, which meant she was horrific. She confessed to not telling her aunt because her aunt would tell the social worker and the social worker would discuss it with her mother. This would make Will's life a living hell. She revealed that Emma and Sarah would feel betrayed if she went home, as if their courage to tell was wasted on her. But they were safe in Oklahoma with another aunt and uncle. They didn't need Elizabeth to keep them safe. Will, Rachel, and Ruthie did.

The counselor left her chair to sit beside Elizabeth. Then Auntie came through the door.

After taking Elizabeth home, Aunt Sheila gave her an aspirin for her headache, tucked her into bed, kissed her forehead, and then smoothed her bangs away from her face. Elizabeth fell into a deep sleep.

* * *

Hours later she awakened into a peaceful silence. Her limbs felt heavy and warm, as if they had been warmed by the sun. Oddly refreshed, she realized her eyelashes were moist, and raised her hands to wipe her eyes. She must have been crying in her sleep.

In her dreamlike state, a thought came to her. Maybe Jesus had orchestrated her escape from her mother for a time, perhaps to strengthen her enough—enough to go home and protect her brother and sisters. He had even ensured her safety by rendering her mother powerless over her—after all, with her father in jail, there could be no back rubs, no extra turns, and no barn.

Fully awake now, she sat up in bed and recalled the story of Samuel from the Bible. The Lord had come to Samuel while he was sleeping. And although God had never intervened in her life like this before, there could be no other explanation. Her dilemma had been resolved as she slept, and the answer was crystal clear: Will and the girls needed her. She was being called to be their protector, and she would not let them down.

THIRTY-SEVEN

Documents

"I went to see the attorney," I begin. "Thanks for getting me her name."

"You're welcome." Maureen replies, pointing at my lap. "I see you have quite a stack of papers."

I'm holding the five-inch stack of papers in my lap. "The attorney thinks I *may* have a case based on a new-memory statute of limitations, but she needed more information, like the transcripts from Dad's first trial. So I went and got them from the courthouse in Charlotte." I pat the stack with my palm. "It's just an hour drive from here."

"Wow, Liz!" Maureen interjects.

"I know, that's how I felt, too. I never knew the trial transcripts were a matter of public record. My past was on this piece of microfilm that someone printed out for fifteen dollars.

"And I sat right there in the parking lot at the courthouse and read the whole thing. I think I was there for almost an hour. There were interviews, trial dates, and trial proceedings. Some of what I read shocked me."

Maureen clasps her hands together and then rests them on her lap. "Shocking?"

"Stunning. See, first I read Emma's statement to the detective, and that was fifteen pages long. Then I came across Sarah's statement, and that was shorter, a page or two. Then I turned the page expecting to see my dad's statement, but instead, I found me."

"You found you?" Maureen asks.

My trembling hands lift up the top few pages and remove a paper-clipped batch of papers. I turn the top document sideways toward Maureen.

"I found *my* interview, the one I never knew I had. I mean, I knew a little of it. But the slides of that memory were pretty blank, and I didn't know those slides were recorded. But it was the interview I thought I'd botched because of my stuttering. The one I thought was no good. See? Here I am: Elizabeth Luther, White Female, Date of Birth: 2-16-65. It's five pages long, and I don't remember it."

"Liz, this is amazing," she murmurs.

"And remember I told you I thought I'd said something about Halloween, but I couldn't remember what I'd said? It's right here." Breathless, I point to the transcripts and the word *Halloween*. "And the reason I told the detective I remembered this particular time was because it was going to be my last time to trick-or-treat. I've never told anyone that except you, Maureen. But I told Detective Sims the same thing."

Turning to the third page of another document, I point to a portion of the transcript I've starred, circled with a pen, and then highlighted with a yellow marker.

"And the best part's here," I point, my voice an octave higher as I read. "'And the People have also agreed—we have knowledge of possibly a third offense—a third, separate case.' The case number in this trial transcript is the same case number on my interview page. The case numbers match. *I* am the third case. I *was* like Emma and Sarah. I *was* part of the plea bargain. I *was* strong back then."

"Liz, how validating for you," she murmurs, now leaning back in her chair. "And yes, you were always strong. You are a survivor."

THIRTY-EIGHT

Strategy

Elizabeth revealed to Aunt Sheila that she had decided to go home. Aunt Sheila was supportive, even while she reminded Elizabeth she needn't rush her return.

Even so, Elizabeth was preparing herself for her return home. Every day she attended school she didn't take academic notes, she was taking what she considered life notes. She wrote out numerous scenarios, screenplays replete with characters, scenes and orchestrated dialogue. Page after page after page filled her binder. She knew she had to be prepared for the unexpected and to do this, she must get inside her mother's head.

The first scene revealed a telephone call listing specific demands using a selected vocabulary and a star, highlighted in yellow that read, *act like you don't give a damn. Heavy sigh, don't respond*

208

at all, silence makes mom uneasy. Subsequent scenes included her return trip to Michigan, beginning with the moment she spotted her mother at the gate.

Her mother was unpredictable, so Elizabeth composed a number of mini plays to address a wide range of variables.

She watched the bullies at school and recognized many of her mother's characteristics. She'd been away from home long enough to recognize that her mother was nothing more than an adult bully. Her mother had no clout with God and in fact, violated the ways of the loving God she had learned about through Aunt Sheila.

Elizabeth also found that she could present with a sense of superiority and apathy that unsettled both students and teachers. She practiced rolling her eyes, or better yet, narrowing her eyes to near-slits then blinking once very slowly. She practiced speaking through clenched teeth, which allowed her to appear angrier than she felt. Elizabeth felt a new sense of power and found she stuttered less, too.

Monday arrived, and the telephone rang. Per her script, she began by disregarding basic civilities and ignoring her mother's hello.

"You need to know that if I choose to come home, I'm not seeing Dad," she dictated, amazed at her fluency. "You ask me to see him once, and I'll be on the next plane back to Colorado."

"You have my word," her mother assured her.

"I don't want your word. I want to be clear."

"Okay," her mother placated.

"And a lock on my bedroom door."

"Done," said her mother. "Ask Will. All the bedroom doors have locks."

"I'm calling Emma and Sarah whenever I want," she continued.

"Of course. I want you to call them, so you can tell them how things have changed."

"If you lay one hand on me or anyone, I'll kick your ass. And then I'll go to the nearest police station and take the kids with me."

The looming silence jarred Elizabeth, and she wondered if she'd gone too far.

"The church made me do that," her mother sniffed. "That's why we don't go to church anymore."

Elizabeth took care to hide her relief.

"You have my word," said her mother.

"I don't care about your word, but I'll give coming back to Michigan a trial run," Elizabeth interrupted.

"Wait, so you're coming home?" her mother asked.

"I didn't say home, I said a trial run," Elizabeth retorted.

"Okay! I'll call the airline tonight, and you'll be home by tomorrow! Here, tell William!" her mother sang.

"Liz?" the boyish voice whispered.

"I'm coming home," she replied.

"When?" William whispered.

"Tomorrow. I promise."

Hanging up the telephone and retreating to her bedroom, she began packing.

"Remember you're a phone call away," Aunt Sheila spoke from the doorway. "You can always call collect, and we can fly you right back here."

Elizabeth nodded, holding a folded T-shirt. "Will and the girls need me," she said. Sighing, she turned back toward her duffel bag.

"I know," her aunt agreed. "They do need someone, but I'm not sure it's supposed to be you."

"Auntie, I can see how things are. I can let Em and Sarah know if it really is safe to come home," she added.

"That's true, and I won't try to stop you. But I want to tell you two things."

Elizabeth nodded.

"First, I love you. Don't forget that."

"I won't," Elizabeth whispered, her eyes welling with tears.

"Second, don't show any fear around your mom. If she sees you afraid, she wins. She's not the devil. She just wants you to think she is."

Elizabeth nodded.

"Wait! Sorry—three things," Aunt Sheila interjected. "I'd never try to trick you into staying. Your mother manipulates, and I hate that. But can I just say I wish you'd stay and let me love you just a little longer? You don't know it, but you need to be loved."

She reached for her niece, and the two embraced while Elizabeth silently acknowledged her aunt was right.

But the more important truth was that Will, Rachel, and Ruthie needed Elizabeth more than Elizabeth needed her aunt.

THIRTY-NINE

My Old House

After securing the court documents, I decided if there was other evidence to be unearthed, the best place to start would be my old neighborhood.

It had been ten years since I had seen my old house, and cresting what I knew to be the final hill, I took my foot off the accelerator and coasted to the driveway entrance.

As I pull into the semicircular driveway, the house emerges into view. Looming before me it is still old, still gray, and still standing.

Craning my neck out the window and looking toward my father's second-story bedroom window, an eeriness surrounds me. I tuck my head back inside my car as an overwhelming crawling sensation overtakes my arms and legs. I look down, expecting to see bugs or spiders crawling on me, but I see nothing. Perplexed, I

212

realize the sensation is coming from beneath my skin. I scratch my forearms with my fingernails with no relief.

Taking in deep slow breaths, I remind myself why I am here. "There are no bugs or spiders crawling on you," I say aloud in my car. "It just feels like it, but there are no bugs or spiders crawling on you."

Turning away from the house, I look to the right where the faded red, ominous barn emerges before me. The sliding door slopes downward into the earth, hanging by a lone hinge.

Easing around the driveway and farther away from his bedroom window, the crawling sensation eases. I park beneath the still great weeping willow and turn off my car.

In my rearview mirror I see my bangs matted to my forehead, saturated in perspiration. My face is pale, my eyes are wide as saucers. Opening my car door, I notice the now earthen driveway—no gravel. No more crunching or grinding of wheels.

Ever.

The earthy river smell fills my nostrils, and I remember looking for crayfish with Will and Sarah.

I cross the lawn and step up onto the disintegrating concrete porch. Plentiful dandelions emerge from jagged crevices of crumbling cement, bobbing their brilliant yellow tufts in greeting. *We know you.*

I knock on my old door. It opens, and I recognize the occupant as my former neighbor. I introduce myself, and she nods.

"I remember you," she replies. She is neither welcoming nor rude. She is, I determine, uneasy.

I ask if I can take a few minutes to visit my old house.

She hesitates. "It's a mess. I haven't cleaned yet today."

"Please, just a few minutes?" I press.

A brief silence ends with her consenting nod. Before she has opportunity to change her mind, I step inside, knowing I will have to hurry. I find myself standing in our old toy room upon the same green, now threadbare carpeting. Moving forward, I enter the dining room where familiar brown paneling whispers to me. Through the archway and into the kitchen I see the remains of a fractured, green-tiled linoleum floor.

My feet continue moving, and I am at the bottom of the same brown steps leading to my father's bedroom. The crawling sensation returns, but I consider my reluctant hostess and press on, ascending the staircase where all but two steps creak under my weight.

Pausing at the top of the landing, I turn to the left.

His bedroom peers at me, and at the far end I see my white windowsill nestled in place, surrounded by circular, white, raised paint. The familiar walls beckon, and I answer, moving my feet forward, this time willingly entering his chamber. Once inside, the swirls tag me in our childhood game, and as I close my eyes, the humming noise begins. Light and warmth envelop me.

I hesitate.

Opening my eyes I realize I don't want to go away. I don't need to go away. The humming dissipates, and an odd silence accentuates the ordinariness of this room: four walls, a ceiling, floor, and window. Within this room my white wall was conceived, and in this same room I will lay her to rest.

214

Maureen's voice comes to me. "There may come a day when you may not need your white wall…"

Today is that day.

Turning around, descending the steps, I approach the back door, where my hostess awaits. Glancing to my left, the old laundry room flashes an image of Will's eyes before me. My heart constricts, and I cannot breathe. My lungs feel as if they will burst.

I whisper a thank-you, exit the house, and hurry to my car. Once inside, I grasp the steering wheel with both hands and rest my forehead at the apex of the steering wheel. I am not the only child who survived this house. There were six other childhoods lost.

Reaching over to the passenger's side, I rummage in my purse, find my inhaler and take two puffs.

Starting my car, I turn on the air conditioning with trembling hands. My head feels as if it is on fire. I find my aspirin bottle, open it and take two, washing them down with my now warm bottled water. The cool air blasts my face, and what might have been a headache is squelched.

Closing my eyes, I remember my father's sentence for his part of the destruction: six months in jail on a work-release program. Shaking my head back and forth, I lift my head and then reopen my eyes.

Turning out of the driveway, I head for the next gravel road to the left. I have a few more homes to visit.

FORTY

Arrival

Disembarking the plane a little after ten o'clock in the evening, Elizabeth scanned the sparse crowd at the gate area. A woman dressed all in black and sporting platinum-blonde hair forced a smile her way.

Is that my mom? Checking her surprise, Elizabeth strode toward her, and a nonchalant but polite hello comprised their reunion.

On their way to the car, Elizabeth estimated Mom had lost about twenty pounds. She was wearing black eyeliner and peach lip gloss. She was wearing a snug, above-the-knee black skirt and a matching silk blouse casually unbuttoned, revealing cleavage Elizabeth had never noticed before. Her mother looked *available*.

Although her mother appeared different, her aura remained unchanged, and the two walked in silence to the parking garage.

216

Mom directed her to the new, silver Honda, and the two got into the car, shutting their doors simultaneously.

Mom turned toward Elizabeth. The liquid black eyeliner accentuated her narrowing eyes.

"Let's get one thing straight. I'm your legal guardian now. You're not to call anyone unless—"

A guttural scream prefaced Elizabeth's throwing her door wide open, grabbing her duffel bag, and bolting from the car.

"Hey! What?!" Mom yelped, scrambling out of the car in confusion. Spotting her daughter hurrying toward the neon exit sign, she stumbled after her, tripping along in her black heels until she caught up.

"Wait! Please wait!" she panted near the stairwell.

"I knew it!" Elizabeth shouted, defiance echoing throughout the parking garage. "You haven't changed!"

"Wait! I'm sorry! I want you to call your sisters and tell them—"

"I *am* telling them!" she interrupted. "Telling them you *already tried* threatening me not to call. And I'm not just telling them, I'm telling *everyone*: the social worker, the cops, anyone who'll listen!" Looking into her mother's eyes, she snarled, "I will *never* lie for you again."

"I'm not asking you to lie," her mother whined, her trembling hands now hovering around her lips.

"You have before," Elizabeth retorted.

"That's in the past. I'm different now," her mother pled.

"Oh, you keep your word now, Rebecca? We agreed I call who I want, remember?"

"Y-yes, we agreed," her mother acquiesced. "And I said I'm sorry."

"I'm done with sorry," Elizabeth spat. She paused, pleased with the results of using her mother's first name. She had seen a student use this on a teacher and it had been effective then, too.

"But William, the girls, they're waiting. Please can you give me one more chance? For them?"

"Screw with me again, and I'm done," she said through clenched teeth. "Will and the girls have made it this long without me. They'll survive if they have to." Without another word, Elizabeth turned and began the trek back toward the car where both doors still hung open.

The hour-long ride home was silent, and Elizabeth, sensing her mother's uneasiness, did nothing to alleviate it. Pulling into the driveway of their new home, her mother clicked the garage remote, and the door slid upward and open.

"Liz, I just want to say that you have my word: I'll never ask you to lie again, because now there's nothing to lie about."

Elizabeth turned toward her mother, blinked once, sighed slowly, and turned away. When Elizabeth did not reply, her mother reached for her purse and rummaged through it.

"Where's that house key?" she murmured. "Oh, Liz? One little thing: please don't mention to the kids that your dad's in jail. If they ask, tell them we've separated, and he has an apartment in Charlotte while we work things out. And Em and Sarah are on vacation with relatives. You were on vacation, too, and now you're home—oh, here's my keys. Ready?"

Elizabeth opened her car door without reply and wondered if Mom realized she'd already broken her promise by telling her to lie. Whether her mother realized it or not was of no consequence to Liz. Her mother had not changed, and Elizabeth knew who she was dealing with.

She knew who the enemy was.

FORTY-ONE

Old Friends

Summer 1992, twenty-seven years old

Ten minutes later I'm knocking upon their door and I realize Titus and Olivia must be in their seventies by now. The last time I saw them I was sixteen, returning from Cedar Point with their son and daughter-in-law. It was the day Dad had been arrested and taken to jail. It was the day I'd left Will and the girls with Mom and headed for Colorado.

Titus opens the door, and as his gray eyes widen in surprised recognition, he smiles and welcomes me inside. I enter their home and find a frail Olivia seated in a recliner, a crocheted afghan blanketing her. She adjusts the afghan and sits up, smiling in surprise.

"Please," Titus offers, extending his hand toward the couch. "Please have a seat. How are you?"

"Pretty good," I smile. "And you two?"

220

"Still kickin'," Titus replies, chuckling. "Olivia's had some heart troubles, but doing okay now."

"I'm glad you're doing better," I say to Olivia. "I want to, well, first, thank you for seeing me unannounced and all."

"Been a long time," Titus replied.

"It has. Maybe ten years?"

Olivia nods in agreement.

"I just came from the old place," I add.

"Your old neighbors moved in, from what I hear," Titus confirms.

"Yes. The lady let me walk around inside, kind of a going-back-in-time journey for me. Some things are hard to remember though."

"That's understandable," Olivia offers. "Bet there's a lot you'd like to forget."

I nod again.

"I was wondering—do you remember much about the day my dad was arrested?"

Titus pauses and glances at Olivia.

"Well, you know it was Tom, my brother, who led your dad to Christ, right?"

I nodded.

"So the day your dad was arrested, Tom went straight away to the jail to see him. We were all so shocked, 'Lizabeth—so shocked it was almost too hard to take—and Tom, well, he said he just had to talk to your dad himself, face to face. So he went straight to the jail, and we just couldn't believe it when your dad admitted he'd been molesting you girls…"

I freeze in my place on the couch, my mouth suddenly parched.

"Dad admitted it?" I ask thickly.

Titus nodded, leaning forward, his great, aged hands clasped together as he closed his eyes, shaking his gray head back and forth sorrowfully. "Sure did. Admitted it from his own cell, same day he was arrested. Told Tom he had a problem and needed help. That's why Tom posted his bond. My brother never forgave himself after he found out your dad changed his story in court. Stood there and said you girls was makin' it all up."

I am quiet, still trying to absorb that my father *admitted* he molested us.

"You know, 'Lizabeth," Olivia began. "After your father was arrested, I remembered this time I was at your house. You might remember it—you came down your parents' bedroom stairs, holding your hands out in front of you—and you said the strangest thing about needing to wash your hands. I asked you why, and you said you'd just given your father a back rub." she paused.

I shake my head. "I don't remember, but I believe you."

"After your dad was arrested I could see it, plain as day. But back then…" her voice trailed off.

"My parents fooled a lot of people," I reply.

"That they did," Titus replied.

"Olivia," I said, "would you be willing to tell an attorney about that, what you remember about me holding out my hands?"

She glanced toward her husband, and he nodded his consent. I gave them my attorney's card, and thanking them, I left.

The clock in my car revealed I'd been in their home a mere fifteen minutes. In a quarter of an hour I'd discovered my father had admitted to sexually abusing all of us. And I'd already found a witness who saw me holding out my hands, on my way to wash them, after giving Dad a back rub.

Traveling less than a mile down the road to the home of Margaret and Randy Foster, my parents' former best friends, I knock twice and the door opens.

"Hello," I say.

"No, thanks, I don't need anything," Margaret says.

"No, I'm not selling anything. I'm Liz—used to be Liz Luther."

"'Lizabeth?" she asks in surprise.

I nod.

Her eyes scan my face for just a moment. "Oh, my goodness! Of course it's you. Please," and she ushers me in, closes the door, then takes both of my hands in a tender gesture. "How are you?" she asks.

"I'm well," I reply. "I was wondering, could I talk with you for a few minutes? And Randy? I m-mean, if he's home?"

"My heavens, of course," she murmurs. "Here, make yourself at home." She pulls out a chair from her dining room table and gestures me to sit in it. "Randy's downstairs, I'll go down and let him know you're here."

Moments later she returns with a glass of lemonade and her husband Randy at her side.

"'Lizabeth?" Randy greets me with the same gentle smile I remember from my youth. He reaches down and pats my shoulder as he walks around the dining table and sits across from me. Margaret sits adjacent both of us, on the end.

I smile. Titus and Olivia were Margaret's parents as well as Doug's parents. Her world at one time had been very small, almost too close knit.

"Thank you for seeing me," I begin. "I just came from your folks' house." I pause. "R-R-Randy?" I look down at the bits of lemonade pulp floating in my glass. "Back when we all went to Wheaton Road, Dad t-told me that you and Lois touched each other, too, and kept it a secret. I know this is an awkward question, but—"

"'Lizabeth," Randy clears his throat. "If I ever had those feelings for my own daughter, I couldn't live with myself. Delbert's a sick man. He's also a liar. And it sickens me he would even use my name."

I close my eyes as his words soothe my soul. I hadn't realized until now that, short of hearing this from Randy himself, I would have gone to my grave believing what my father had told me over and over again.

"Th-thank you. It helps me to hear you say that." My voice trembles. I inhale and continue. "And…c-can I ask one more thing? Does anything strange about my family stand out to you now? In hindsight, I mean?"

Margaret nods, turns toward Randy, then back to me. "About a month before Delbert was arrested, I had spoken to Randy and my dad about your dad falling away from the faith. I'd noticed he missed a lot of Wednesday night services. One of you older girls stayed home with him at least every other Wednesday night. I'd ask one of your brothers or sisters where you were, and someone would always say you had to stay home because your dad had a headache." Margaret stops and purses her lips. She looks down and then takes a sip of lemonade. She sets the glass back on the table and clears her throat. "And after Del was arrested, I saw it. But at the time, the idea that he was molesting you girls? Well, it never crossed my mind."

"Would you mind sharing that with my attorney?" I ask.

"Of course, if it will help."

I give her my attorney's card.

The silence that follows is not uncomfortable as I finished my lemonade. As a child I'd been so familiar with their home, I would've rinsed my glass and placed it on the top shelf of their dishwasher. But my childhood days had passed.

Thanking them, I stand, leaving my glass on the table.

They walk me to the door, and Margaret reaches for me. I realize I am embracing a mother who never sent her daughter to be molested. Tears well up in my eyes as I realize how much she must love Lois. Randy presents his open arms in invitation, and I know I am going to hug a man who has never molested his daughter.

It is as if I've met them both for the first time.

Driving away, my heart still full, I consider that I could be like them. I could, perchance, love a little girl. Maybe I should tell Matt that.

Back on the highway, I know I have one more stop to make—Tom Kearny's house. If my father confessed to Tom, his testimony would be invaluable. Arriving in less than five minutes, I get out, knock on his door, and wait. No one answers. There is no car in the driveway.

Disappointed but not dissuaded, I call him later that evening.

"'Lizabeth, your father promised he'd get help. I'd never have bailed him out otherwise. Ask your brother, Todd, I told him Delbert admitted everything to me."

"I believe you," I reply. "Would you mind talking with my attorney about what Dad told you?" I ask.

He agrees, and after thanking him, I hang up.

I slump into the chair at my kitchen table, exhausted. In one day I have secured three witnesses.

I can't wait to see Maureen.

FORTY-TWO

Visitor

Elizabeth took great care observing her new home environment. She was scheduled to talk on the phone with Em and Sarah on Saturdays, and she needed to tell them if it was indeed safe for them to come home.

She learned the details of her father's sentence that included six months of jail time on a work-release program. This meant her father lived at the jail except for when he went to work and back, allowing him to keep his job and ensure he was supervised. He had to submit his time cards at the end of every week, detailing his arrival and departure times.

Dad was allowed supervised visits with Will, Rachel, and Ruth at a restaurant near the jail for one hour each Friday after work. Elizabeth was incredulous to learn her mother was the "supervisor" during these visits. That the same woman who'd sent her upstairs for years to give Dad back rubs was now charged with the safekeeping of three minor children was sickening.

At least Elizabeth didn't have to go see him. Instead, each Friday she came home to a quiet, empty house. After fixing some dinner, she'd go to her room and listen to the radio or read until Will and the girls got home.

Her father was also allowed one-hour telephone privileges from his jail cell Monday through Thursday evenings. There were no phone privileges on Friday nights, since he was allowed to visit his family at the restaurant.

Monday through Thursday followed a predictable routine. Elizabeth, Will, and her two younger sisters rode the bus to and from school each day. After school, they did their homework as their mother prepared dinner.

At five o'clock, their mother's bottle of cherry liqueur made its way onto the kitchen counter alongside the evening meal preparations. Dinner was served at five forty-five, buffet style. The food remained in the pots on the stove, and the children helped themselves and ate together in front of the television.

Mom topped off her glass and headed for her bedroom, waiting for Dad to call from jail at six o'clock. At first, Mom took great care to close her bedroom door during the phone calls. Over time, however, her vigilance eased and, especially after ingesting two glasses of liqueur, she would stroll into her bedroom, leaving the door slightly ajar. Portions of the conversation filtered into the den where the children were watching television as they ate their evening meal.

Elizabeth sat in the recliner closest to the bedroom door.

"I told them I had to change attorneys because the first one was incompetent," her mother slurred. "Yeah, the divorce process starts over. Before it gets to the final stage, all the girls will be home. No, once they're home, they're ours to keep. No, they have a different worker now and this one hasn't talked to Liz since she got home. No, not even a phone call, no school visits, nothing. Shows you how bad of a parent I am, doesn't it? The bitch just calls me once a month and asks me how it's going, and of course it's going fine. I tell her I'm making *progress* bonding with my own daughter thanks to the *skills* I've learned," she scoffed. "Sarah? Her hearing is next week. I'm still calling her on Saturdays, and Liz tells her everything is good. I know because I'm listening on the other end. No, she's not encouraging her to come home, but she's not discouraging her either. No, I can't tell Liz to tell Sarah to come home. Because she's changed, Del. She's not the same kid. She's mouthy, doesn't even stutter any more either. God, no! I don't think it'd help if you talked to her. I know you used to be close. *Used to be*, Del. She won't even come see you on Fridays. If I made her talk to you, she'd call that bitch Sheila and be on the next flight to Colorado. No, I'll get Sarah back, or there'll be hell to pay. My worker is recommending Sarah's return based on what she calls my 'substantial progress,'" she continued sarcastically. "As if she has the right to tell me I'm ready to raise my own kids."

Each telephone conversation revealed new information, and although Elizabeth realized her mother's claim to divorce her father was a ruse, as long as there were no back rubs and no barn, she considered it was safe enough for her sisters to return. There were no drunken outbursts, and there had been no discipline to speak of. No, it wasn't the Cleaver family, but it wasn't the old Luther family, either.

The Friday before Sarah's custody hearing, Elizabeth got off the bus at four fifteen to find Will, Rachel, and Ruth watching television.

"You're not visiting Dad?" she asked William.

"No," he replied. "Mom picked us up from school and then went to get pizza. She said we're eating here tonight."

By six o'clock, however, there was no pizza, and the four children were hungry. With no sign of their mother, Elizabeth prepared to make grilled cheese sandwiches. As she pulled the bread from the pantry, she heard the front door open.

Her mother entered holding a large pizza box and a two-liter soda bottle. She called the children downstairs to the family room and handed them slices of pizza on paper plates.

"Hey guys, I need you to eat down here in front of the old television tonight, not the new one up in the den."

"You told us not to eat in here because of the new couch," Will reminded Mom.

"I know, but just for tonight. Be careful, and keep your drinks on the kitchen counter so they won't spill. Liz? Sorry I'm late. Thanks for starting dinner, but we're good. I need to talk with you up in my room," she said. "Just leave the bread on the counter."

Elizabeth, irritable and hungry, sighed.

"It won't take long," her mother coaxed. "I'll be up in a second. I forgot my purse in the car."

Elizabeth grabbed a pizza slice on her way up the steps and entered her mother's bedroom with the lights still off.

Walking toward the windows, she peered through the curtains into the dusky horizon as she took a bite of pizza. In the autumn sky the moon was already visible, and Elizabeth, curious, watched as her mother walked the length of the driveway. She still didn't have her purse. Was she getting the mail? Her mother stopped at the end of the driveway and looked both ways, then turning around, she headed back toward the house without opening the mailbox. Had she been drinking already? Elizabeth didn't remember smelling any alcohol on her breath as she'd passed her in the kitchen.

Still watching through the curtains, she saw her mother approach the car and open the back door. The dome light illuminated the backseat, where a blue blanket rose up and then slipped away.

It was her father.

Elizabeth gasped. As if in slow motion, Elizabeth's pizza slipped from her hands and fell, landing upside down on the floor.

Frozen in place, she watched Dad quickly turn off the dome light, look around suspiciously, exit the car, and under the cover of a shadowy autumn dusk, slip inside the house.

Nauseous, she steadied herself against the wall. She had not prepared for this. The back rubs were going to happen again.

Moments later, her mother opened the bedroom door abruptly and turned on the light switch. "Oh, clever. So you know he's here," she began curtly. "Your father has something he needs to say to you," she said, ushering him inside. "Del, I told the guard you're working overtime, and Mike said he'd clock you out two hours late. We've got five minutes," she directed, holding up her right hand with her fingers outstretched.

Then she left the room.

Dad approached the bed and sat down, patting the mattress, directing Elizabeth to sit beside him. As if entranced, she obeyed, sitting down to his right.

The moment the mattress squeaked, the humming noise began in her head. His scent of body odor and oil from the car factory assaulted her nostrils, and she reminded herself to be still. She should be very quiet and very still.

He laid his head upon her shoulder, crying. His breath still smelled like coffee, and he was unshaven. He was at least ten pounds thinner.

"I love you," he sniffled, sliding close to her, encircling her shoulder with his right arm. Her body's muscles remembered what to do, and she leaned into him. A crawling sensation overcame her, and she looked down at her legs, surprised there were no bugs on her.

"You've always been my favorite," he whisper-sobbed. "I don't know why things turned out this way. The world just doesn't understand. We gotta get our family back together again, don't we?"

She reminded herself not to move.

"Your mother is going crazy, Liz. She's drinking every night. She's broken up inside, missing Sarah. So when you talk to Sarah tomorrow, can you tell her to come home?" he beseeched. "The hearing is next week, and I don't know what your mother will do if Aunt Suzanne gets to keep her. I think it will push her right over the edge. She's been through a lot, and she just can't take much more. Lizzie?"

Elizabeth stared straight into the white wall and nodded her head.

"Good girl," he praised. Wiping his nose on his sleeve he eyed the clock on the nightstand. "Shit, I gotta go. You head on downstairs, and I'll sneak out behind you. The other kids can't see me—they'd talk. You'll keep our secret, right?"

Standing without a word, she exited the bedroom. Descending the stairs, she saw her mother guarding the entryway.

"I'm taking him back," she whispered.

"I g-g-get that," Elizabeth replied, still unnerved.

"To the jail, I mean," her mother replied haltingly.

From behind her, her father descended the steps and joined his wife. Elizabeth moved aside and watched over her shoulder as her parents quietly exited the screen door and back into the night. Once she heard the car start, she ventured to the door and watched her mother back the car out of the driveway. They were gone. No one had seen them.

She turned to the right and entered the lower level where her brother and sisters were still eating pizza on the new couch in front of the old television. Time had remained unchanged for them. Had she really seen her father with her own eyes? She passed her siblings and went to her bedroom realizing how lucky she had been. This time her father had only five minutes. No one could give a back rub in five minutes.

But next time he might have an hour.

And everyone knew an hour was just enough time.

FORTY-THREE

Mediation

Summer 1992, twenty-seven years old

It was a little over a year since the day we filed the civil suit, and today was the day I was to meet my attorney at the courthouse for a mediation hearing.

Waiting at the courthouse, I'm glad I asked Matt not to come.

"If the recommendation isn't in my favor, I'm going to need some time to deal with that," I'd explained to him. At this point in my marriage, I'd worked hard to establish a sense of dignity. I will take care to protect this and, knowing myself the way I do, if the members of the mediation panel find in favor of Dad, I know I will be an emotional train wreck. I will need some time, a few hours at least, to get myself back on track.

Dad's attorney, Frank Richton, is the same attorney who represented Dad when I was sixteen. Within the past year, Richton had filed numerous motions, although each had been resolved in my favor.

Richton had tried dismissing the case, claiming the statute of limitations had run out. It had, in fact, not run out; based on the new statute of limitations in Michigan, I had one year from the time I experienced a new memory to file a civil claim against the perpetrator. The memory occurred when I was camping with Matt in September of 1990, and I filed my claim the following March— well within the allotted timeframe.

Richton also tried to dismiss the case, claiming that any sexual abuse allegations were untrue. In order to counter this, Sarah agreed to be a co-plaintiff with me because Dad had admitted he molested Sarah as part of his plea agreement in 1981. His own words would convict him.

My attorney pokes her head in through the door of the hall where I'm sitting.

"How are you doing, Liz?"

I smile. "Okay. Any news?"

She shakes her head. "I'll let you know. They've been in there about two hours, so I'm estimating another hour. Do you want to go get some coffee? If they make a decision sooner, I'll meet you right back here."

I shake my head. "No, thanks. I'll just wait."

The least surprising motion Richton filed was the one where Dad claimed he had no memory of the incidents. I was not so afraid of this claim because I'd heard it before and knew now how ludicrous it sounded. It also looked weak on paper when we provided the original transcripts from 1981 revealing Dad remembered the incident with Sarah. We also submitted the names of three witnesses: Olivia, who saw me leaving Dad's bedroom and saying I needed to wash my hands; Margaret, who remembered the numerous Wednesdays nights Dad missed at church and that one of us older girls had to stay home with him each time; and, Tom, the man visited Dad in jail when Dad admitted to molesting all three of us.

I chuckle to myself as I wonder what Dad's face looked like when he saw those three familiar names on our rebuttal list: a former minister, a minister's wife, and the man who baptized him into the faith.

Time passes, and I wonder why I'm not allowed to meet the people on the mediation panel or hear them deliberate. I know from my attorney that the panel is comprised of three individuals with legal expertise. Their job is to review all the evidence from both sides and make a recommendation. Neither side has to accept the recommendation, but my attorney says she's confident our case is solid. She also reminded me there are no guarantees.

I am nervous. Will they believe me?

Forty minutes later, the door at the end of the hallway opens again, and my attorney smiles as she walks toward me. She is holding a lone piece of paper with typed words upon it.

I stand and meet her halfway.

"Good news," she announces, her voice reverberating in the hallway.

"Did they believe us?" I ask.

"I would say one hundred thousand dollars means they believe you." She smiled.

"What?!"

"Each," she interjects. "One hundred thousand dollars, *each*."

She shares the crisp, white paper between us, and as I read the document, I see the word "unanimous."

"It was unanimous? All three of them believed us?"

"All three," she confirms.

I stare at the declaration. "It's like David and Goliath," I murmur, savoring the victory. "What did Dad say?" I ask, grinning.

"He rejected the panel's recommendation, but you and I discussed that earlier and we knew he'd do that, so that's no surprise."

I laugh. "His retirement wages would be garnished until he was six feet under, and he's not about to let that happen. So what's our next step?"

"The trial," she said. "We'll get a date from the judge, serve the subpoenas to our witnesses, and finish this."

FORTY-FOUR

Crazy

Elizabeth hoped her hesitancy on the telephone was obvious to Sarah during their Saturday call.

She knew it was no longer safe for Sarah to come home. If her parents could sneak her dad into the house without anyone knowing, who knew what else they were capable of?

Tuesday arrived, and Elizabeth knew it was the day of the hearing. She acted as if she did not know, and went to school with her sisters as usual. Fourteen-year-old Will stayed home with a low-grade fever.

During her last hour English class, there was a brief knock upon the classroom door. The office helper appeared, holding a pink slip, excusing Elizabeth to take an emergency telephone call in the office.

"Will?" she said, turning away from the school secretary.

"Sorry to call you at school, but Mom's gone nuts. You gotta come home," he whispered.

"What?" she asked, "What do you mean?"

"Just listen. I'll hold up the phone so you can hear."

In the background, a screeching wail rose and fell. "Goddamn those bitches! My Sarah!"

Elizabeth's heart congealed as nausea swept over her.

"Ya hearing that?" he whispered, his voice choking.

"I'm on my way," she replied, trying to sound confident.

Arranging a ride with a schoolmate and arriving home in less than twenty minutes, she eased inside the house through the garage entryway. She stood on the foyer landing. Low moans echoed through the walls from the family room to her right, beyond the closed foyer door.

It was quiet for a moment, then Elizabeth saw Will padding down the stairs from the upstairs den.

"Maybe she's done?" she whispered to him.

A guttural, low growling sound emerged from behind the door, and William shook his head back and forth.

"She's just getting started," he whispered, his chin trembling. "I can't take this shit anymore. She went to court today, and Sarah isn't coming home," he reported.

Another moan filled the air, and Will's trembling palm rose to the crown of his head as he flattened his brown hair down toward his eyes.

"Okay," Elizabeth whispered. "Go on upstairs and watch for the bus. When the girls get home, take them upstairs. I'll deal with Mom."

She waited until she heard Will's bedroom door close. Next, Elizabeth opened the entryway door, determined to meet her mother head on. Turning the corner toward the cacophony, she froze.

She was sitting on her knees upon the blue shag carpet, eyes squinted shut, a stream of tears flowing down her face.

"Goddamn them allllll!" she shrieked.

The rhythmic moaning gradually rescinded, and Elizabeth watched Mom lower herself onto her forearms, rubbing her elbows, raw and bloody, back and forth on the carpet in a slow, sick rhythm.

Liz closed the door. The latch clicked.

Her mother raised her head at the sound. Pushing herself up with her palms, her rocking slowed to a stop, and she cocked her head toward Elizabeth.

"Look who's here," she cackled, waving. "It's my whore-daughter. Hello, whore!" She stopped waving and wiped the snot from her nose with the back of her hand. "You know I never loved you, right? Who could love such an ugly little slut?"

She wiped her chin with her shoulder. "I'm not your father, you know," she said, lowering her chin and peering at Elizabeth beneath raised eyebrows. "I have an *excellent* memory. After this is over and I say"—her mother lowered voice in mockery—"I'm sorry, I didn't know what I was doing, I don't remember. I was taking pills." She laughed hysterically. "Know this, you stupid bitch: I'm *not* sorry. I know what I'm saying, and who I'm saying it to. I *never* loved you, and I *never* will."

"Whatever," Elizabeth attempted, feigning apathy and rolling her eyes. "Come on, Mom, cut the—"

"Don't!" her mother began, rising onto her knees and shrieking. "Don't ever call me Mom again, you little whore!"

Elizabeth took a quick step toward the door.

"Tell me. What did you like more?" she began. "Fucking him or telling the goddamn police on me? How could you?" she screamed, rocking the walls. "I am your mother!"

Leaning forward, her mother began sobbing, beating her right fist on the carpet.

Elizabeth took another step toward the door and, opening it, reached around the doorknob to the other side, turning it to the lock position. Leaving the door ajar in case she needed to make a quick exit, she walked the few steps to the telephone.

Lifting the receiver off the black box she dialed the number for the jail. It was taped to the calendar near the telephone. She asked to speak with her father, and when the male voice decreed it wasn't the inmate's scheduled call time, she paused.

"It's an emergency. Just for a second, please," she pleaded.

After a lengthy wait, her father answered.

"What?" he asked abruptly. "What?"

"Mom didn't get Sarah," Elizabeth said.

"I know. Do you—" her father began.

"She's crazy," Elizabeth interrupted him.

"What?" he asked in irritation.

"Here, listen," she said, holding the receiver toward her screaming mother.

"Sheila and Suzanne—bitches! Goddamn them! Just wait and see if their children come up missing! What goes around comes around!" she shouted, her eye again catching Elizabeth. "Hang up the phone, you whore!" she screamed.

"Ya hearing that?" Elizabeth asked.

"I hear it." He choked.

"If I call the police—" she began.

"God no! They'll take all of you away," said her father. He paused. "Wait! Call Tom and Katherine from the church—call them."

"From the old church?" Elizabeth asked.

"Yeah, Tom will come. The guard is saying—" A click confirmed her father's call was terminated.

Tuning out her mother's babblings, Elizabeth dialed information and got the Kearney's number. Just as her father promised, Tom and Katherine agreed to come.

Hanging up the phone, she ignored her mother's screaming and focused on exiting calmly. Taking care to close the door behind her, she locked her mother in on the main floor. Ascending the stairs she watched out the window with William until the school bus dropped off Rachel and Ruth. Elizabeth met them at the garage-door entrance and led them upstairs, where William had turned on the television. Forty minutes later, the downstairs door creaked open, and two sets of footsteps shuffled inside. Elizabeth descended the stairs to see Tom and Katherine standing side-by-side in the entryway.

Low, rhythmic moans hummed through the main door.

"Mom went to court today and didn't get Sarah," she said, unlocking and opening the door. "Mom's in there."

Tom went first, and Katherine followed closely.

As Rebecca came into full view, Katherine gasped.

Elizabeth's mother looked up. "Well," she croaked, "look who's here! The hypocrites. Hi, hypocrites!" she announced, waving her soiled, bloodied hand.

A panicked silence filled the air.

"Cat got your tongue?" she quipped when no one replied. "Cat's got their tongue." She lowered her head and repeated to the carpet. "Cat's got their tongue—"

"'Lizabeth," Tom commanded, unnerving Elizabeth's mother, who fell silent. "We'll need some clean clothes for your mother. And some towels."

Elizabeth darted upstairs retrieving towels, a washcloth, and a change of her mother's clothing, then hurried back down.

Katherine took the clothing and towels from Elizabeth and took a step toward Elizabeth's mother.

Rebecca looked up and smoothed her hair down with her fingers. Glaring at the three standing in the kitchen, she tucked her legs beneath her now soiled skirt.

"Get the hell out of my house," she spat, "or I'll call the police!"

Katherine hesitated.

Tom marched toward Elizabeth's mother, and Elizabeth watched Mom cower beneath his gaze.

"We'll be the ones calling the police," he declared. "And then you'll learn to live with losing all of your children. Is that what you want, Becky?" he charged.

From behind Elizabeth, Rachel turned the doorknob and poked her head inside.

"What's wrong with Mom, now?" she asked irritably. "We're getting hungry—"

Elizabeth ushered her away from the door and into the foyer, closing the door behind them.

"If this is about Sarah, I say who cares," Rachel said. "We're doing fine without her. We can't help it if she's off living with our rich relatives."

"Guess who I am?" said Ruth, now sitting on the top step, leaning against the wall, banging her head and lolling her eyes.

"We know. You're Mom," Rachel smiled.

"That's not funny," Elizabeth replied.

"Ya gotta laugh, Liz," Will said, appearing beside Ruth. "When she does this crap, there's nothing else you can do."

"She's done this before?" Elizabeth asked

All three nodded.

"It's an act," Will said. "Whenever she doesn't get her way, she does this shit. If she didn't gross me out so much, I'd slap it out of her." He shivered in disgust. "But I'm not touching her."

"Well, let's go upstairs." Elizabeth sighed. "Tom and Katherine are here, so she's fine for now."

The downstairs grew quiet, and about an hour later the entry door opened. Tom appeared, and Elizabeth followed him downstairs.

"Hurry if you can. We're starving," Will called out.

Back in the family room, Elizabeth saw two towels covering a large area on the carpet. Someone had sprayed what smelled like an entire can of disinfectant spray. Her mother sat on the couch in clean clothes, her hair still wet from a shower. Katherine was emptying a bucket of water into the toilet.

"Liz," her mother began in a raspy, tired voice. "I didn't handle your sister not coming home so good. Sorry."

"Mmm," Elizabeth replied, "I'll let the kids know they can come down and eat?"

"Forgive me?" her mother pressed.

"Sure," Elizabeth replied hollowly.

Katherine set the now empty bucket on the kitchen floor.

"That's a good note to leave on, I think?" she said to her husband.

"I agree," he replied.

"Thanks for coming," Elizabeth said, following them to the door.

"Yes, thank you," Mom's voice called from the couch.

"You're welcome," Tom shouted. He then looked at Elizabeth and touched her arm. "Call anytime," he whispered. "I'm glad we were home."

"Me, too," she whispered, giving his forearm a squeeze, "Me, too."

FORTY-FIVE

Nightmare

"I'm not sleeping well," I begin. "The same nightmare wakes me up every night. I think all these trial delays from Dad's lawyer are stressing me out."

"How long ago did you start the proceedings?"

"Summer, 1992," I say. "That's a lot of delays."

"It is. Can you tell me about your nightmare?" Maureen asks.

"I'm running from Dad and Todd—they're chasing me, holding a black body bag. I try screaming for help, but my lips are sewn shut with black thread. Twice last week they got me, zipped me up in it, and dumped me in a river. Then, other times, I break open the seam on my lips and scream so loud I wake myself up before they get me."

"Do you remember what you're feeling when you are in your nightmare?"

I pause. "Terror. They're trying to kill me, and I can't scream for help. And if I do scream, no one's around to hear me. We're in some kind of isolated, wooded area."

"So you're feeling terrified, and you can't scream for help. What do you think it could mean?"

"I don't know," I hesitate. "It could mean I'm still afraid of Dad and Todd? Or—maybe this court case will stress me out and I'll revert to that old state of terror I felt as a kid—when I couldn't talk? I've been through that kind of fear, almost takes the skin off you."

"So you could still be afraid of your dad and Todd, and/or you worry you'll end up in that place where you were terrified and were unable to speak, like during the first trial?"

"Yes, and now that we're talking about it, I think I'm afraid of Dad. Todd is just Dad's lackey. If it were only Todd in my dream, I think I'd try to take him out. But Dad is looming and scary," I shudder a little. "He's tall and loud—in real life, too. He's terrifying."

"Your dad is looming and massive," she probes, "so is he an adult in your dream or bigger than an adult?"

"An adult, the same size he is now."

"And in your dream, are you the same size as you are now?"

I hesitate. "No. I'm about nine or ten."

"Then in your nightmare you feel terror in the context of when you were a little girl?"

I try piecing it together. "Maybe I'm remembering the terror I felt as a child?"

"Perhaps. Let me ask, are you around the same size as your dad, I mean in real time, not dream time?"

"He outweighs me by about fifty pounds, but I'm a few inches taller than him."

"And you said you might be feeling stressed out by the trial delays. Have you thought about how you might feel when you see him at the trial?"

"Not yet." I pause. "But maybe I'm afraid that at this trial I'll feel the same terror I did when I was sixteen."

"So in your dream, you're in that childhood place where adults appear big?"

"Yes. But sitting here in the daylight, I don't think I'll revert to that same childhood place where I can't speak. I mean, I don't think it's possible. I'm madder now." I sigh. "Do you think talking about the nightmare will make it stop?"

"It might. But if it doesn't, some people can bring themselves out of a nightmare by talking to the people in the nightmare. If you could talk to this terrified little girl, what would you say to her?"

"I'd grab ahold of her and tell her not to be afraid because I'd keep her safe. I'd promise to protect her. And that whoever is chasing her will be made very sorry."

"Now substitute the word *I*…" Maureen reminds me.

"Okay," I begin, organizing my thoughts. "I have no reason to be afraid because I can keep myself safe. I can protect myself. And I'm doing all I can to make Dad sorry." I hesitate for just a moment. "Do you really think I'll be able to talk to myself in my nightmare? I think that would be awesome."

"You'll have to tell me when we meet next," Maureen replies. "That is, if you have the nightmare again."

"Number two's about the court case. My attorney wants me to think about what I want if Dad wants to negotiate. Matt and I are thinking if we're awarded a substantial amount of money, Dad and Todd would both say Sarah and I did this for the money. Not that I don't want money—I mean, I work for money. I need money. But if Dad is forced to pay us, say by garnishing his wages, until his death?" I shake my head. "I don't think I want to get a check from my dad every month. I don't want to be reminded of him that often."

"That makes sense," Maureen replies.

"And I don't want there to be any question about why I'm doing this. I mean, for Dad and Todd. I want Dad to know that I know what he did. I want Todd to know what Dad did. This kind of abuse can be cyclical. I don't know for sure, but I suspect Dad was abused by his parents."

"That also makes sense," Maureen echoes.

"Matt and I were thinking of asking for some money to help pay for court and therapy expenses. Then I'd like a meeting with Dad to confront him. I don't know how Sarah would feel about that."

"You want to make sure Sarah is comfortable with your requests?"

"She says it's up to me, but I want to be sure."

Maureen is silent.

"Guess I should keep praying about it," I said. "On to number three, I guess. I've wanted to ask your opinion on something. I've been thinking of telling Matt it would be okay if we had children—I mean, a little girl."

Maureen leans back in her chair, her pen still on her end table. "Matt doesn't think it would be okay?"

"Not him. Me. When he asked me to marry him I said I would on one condition: we could never have a daughter. I never wanted to be like my mother. I knew it was possible to hate your own child, because my mother hated me. I was so alone. I was so afraid. The idea of subjecting a child to that kind of loneliness and fear, I never, ever want to do that."

"You are familiar with loneliness and fear. And you don't have any children of your own, so let's look at this from another angle. On the children's unit, do you yell at or hit any of the children?"

"Um, no. I'd be fired." I counter.

"Yes, you would." She smiles. "And do you think it says anything that you choose to work with children every day?"

"I love kids," I say. "There's something spiritual, almost healing about them."

"Do you find yourself making excuses for any of the kids' perpetrators?"

"No way!"

"And didn't you report a teacher for slapping a little boy on the hand?" she asks.

"Yes. I told him he had until shift change to report himself and if he didn't, I would. He never reported it. So he left me no choice."

"So you defended a little child when he could not defend himself."

"I did. Because who am I—or who is anyone—to take out their impatience on a child? That's not the child's fault, that's the adult's. Children are little spirits running around on God's earth, trying to be loved. They don't deserve to be slapped."

"So based on your actions on the children's unit, you *value* children. You've chosen differently than your mother. You've chosen to honor their childhood by protecting them."

In the quietness, a breath of fresh air seems to pass over me.

"By choosing to 'mother' these children this way," Maureen continues, "could you say you've been mothering yourself? Kind of laying the groundwork again after digging up the foundation your mother laid for you?"

"By my actions I'm proving myself a better mother than my mother, though I don't have any children of my own," I say, nodding.

"And you also had your own little girl of sorts in your nightmare. Do you remember what you wanted to tell her?"

"That I'd protect her and keep her safe."

"If we look at these words, these tender, mothering words, what kind of parent do *you* think you'd be to a little girl?"

"The kind of parent I wish I'd had," I said.

"So." Maureen crosses her legs. "Do I think you would be a good mother to a little girl? I'll answer that, if you answer it first."

"I wouldn't be perfect, but I know I'd protect my daughter. I'd love her. I don't think I'd be able to help myself. I would totally, unconditionally love her."

Maureen puts her pen down with certainty. "You're right, Liz. You would."

FORTY-SIX

A Plan

Cherry liqueur in hand, her mother sat on the edge of Elizabeth's bed. "Have some?" she offered, extending her glass.

Elizabeth declined.

"My counselor thought I should share something with you," she said, slurring her words. "Can you put that down for a sec?"

Must be her second glass, Elizabeth thought as she laid the driver's training booklet down on her bed.

"Soon we'll have our old family back—first Emma's coming home, then your dad, then Sarah."

"When?" Elizabeth asked nonchalantly, even as the words, "we'll have our old family back again," cut like razors into her spine.

"A few months at the least, I mean the most," Mom giggled, now lying down on her back, legs dangling over the edge of the bed.

A Plan

"Lawyers are saying your dad should be home by the end of April. He won't be able to be alone in the house with you kids, or drive you kids around unless I'm in the car. That's part of his probation. Hope you'll pass your driver's test next week so you can help with errands," her mother said thickly.

Elizabeth nodded, her mind in overdrive as she counted the steps she'd have to complete to get out of this house before her father came home. She would need an apartment, and of course a driver's license. She needed her own car and a job. The apartment would have to be big enough to share with Will and the girls if necessary.

As her mother babbled, Elizabeth realized the end of April was less than three months away.

* * *

Liz passed her driver's test the following week and also secured a job at the local grocery store, catching rides from friends or, when possible, borrowing her mother's car to get to work and back. Her February birthday afforded her the opportunity to ask for cash in lieu of birthday presents. And rather than a party for her upcoming high school graduation gift in June, she asked her mother for an early graduation cash gift.

"It would help me save for a car, so when Dad gets home, I can help run the kids around," she reminded her mother.

By March, Elizabeth had purchased a black Cutlass for three hundred and fifty dollars. Securing a job at the local grocery store as a bagger, after taxes, she brought home around five dollars an hour. She squirreled her money into a coffee can, hidden under the deck in the backyard.

Keeping her grades up to maintain her volleyball scholarship and Pell Grant eligibility, she continued working as many hours as she could.

An apartment security deposit, one month's rent, and utility hook-ups would run her one thousand dollars. Then, she'd need another seven hundred dollars a month to maintain her independence.

Cheryl, a newly divorced checker at the grocery store, asked Elizabeth if she wanted to share apartment expenses. Elizabeth wavered. She needed her own apartment in case her brother or sisters also needed a place to stay. Politely declining she thanked her for the offer.

The end of April came too soon, and counting out her money, she found she'd saved seven hundred dollars.

And then her father came home.

FORTY-SEVEN

Settlement

I awoke early. Today was the day.

Sarah arrived last night, driving from out of state to be here for the trial.

Matt, Sarah, and I rode to the courthouse together, arriving in the parking lot an hour before schedule. Approaching the steps of the courthouse, Matt held my right hand, and Sarah walked on my left.

Ascending the steps I felt a now-familiar sense of peace and assuredness, not to be confused with victory. I had already won.

Opening the great glass doors and entering the lobby, I take in a deep breath and then exhale as my eyes rest upon the woman standing in the corner of the lobby.

"I can't believe she'd show her face here," I whisper, shaking my head. "I wonder if she'd still be here if I told her she was next."

"Let's find out," Matt suggests.

He walks across the room toward my mother, nods, and begins speaking to her. Her eyes widen beneath her bleached-blond hair, and she clutches her black purse, turns, and exits the building.

The delight that envelops me is intoxicating and infectious as Matt, Sarah, and I all chuckle together upon Matt's return.

"Look, Margaret Foster's over there," Sarah said. "She looks exactly the same to me."

"I just saw Tom Kearney head for the bathroom," I offer. "Can you believe they care enough to testify?"

"I don't see Todd," Matt adds. "And where's your dad's sister, the one who thinks you guys made all this up? What's her name, Veronica?"

"Haven't seen her," said Sarah. "Could they be in another waiting area? I know Dad and Florence are here—at least Dad has to be here—but I don't see him either."

Our attorney enters the foyer wearing a blue suit and modest heels. Smiling, she approaches the three of us.

"Time to head to the courtroom—your father and Richton will come up after we do. I asked them to give us five minutes. Liz? You look like you're holding up okay?"

I nod. She scans the room, and her eyes rest on Margaret.

"I'll let Mrs. Foster and Mr. Kearney know we're headed up to the courtroom."

After greeting Margaret, my attorney motioned for the three of us to follow her, and then waited for us to catch up at the elevator.

"Mrs. Foster's going to wait for Mr. Kearney. Let's go on up, so we don't end up riding in the elevator with Mr. Luther and Mr. Richton," she says, pushing the elevator button.

We enter the elevator, go up two floors, and follow our attorney to a set of wide, oak, swinging double doors. She pushes the right side open, and we enter a large, dimly lit courtroom.

"We're seated on the right," she said.

Of course we are.

"Liz? Sarah? You two will sit with me there," she said, pointing to a rectangular table about ten feet away. Matt, you can sit right here behind us. Um, I hear Richton," she said, turning her ear toward the door and smiling. "I wonder who doesn't hear him. Anyway, your dad has to be close behind, so let's move to our table and out of their path."

There are three chairs at our table. A stack of papers sit staggered on top of it. About ten feet in front of us, a raised stage boasts a great, oak desk for the judge. Empty juror chairs sit alone on my right within a wooden, gated area. On my left and about six feet away is the other rectangular table, the one where Richton and Dad will sit.

From behind me, I hear Richton's voice.

"Here, Delbert, over here on the left," he says loudly.

I turn around and recognize Mr. Richton, Dad's attorney since the first criminal trial, just over ten years ago. Dad follows right behind Richton, as if needing protection. Dad's eyes are fixed upon the floor as he keeps pace with his attorney. I do not look away and hope he will look at me. I am struck by how short Dad is. I turn to Sarah.

"Did he shrink?" I whisper.

"Looks like it," she whispered back.

Gone was the looming, massive monster. In its place stood a puny, wrinkled old man.

"You guys can take a seat," our attorney whispers to us. "I'm going to make sure Margaret and Tom know where to go. You two okay?"

Sarah and I nod at the same time. We turn to sit down as our attorney exits the courtroom to look for our witnesses. I turn my chair to the left so I can still see Dad making his way to his side of the courtroom.

Richton abruptly stops and looks at me.

"You look just like your mother," he barks as if to the whole courtroom.

I raise my eyebrows at him wondering what sort of man chooses to wait until the opposing counsel leaves to address me. I do not move, and my eyes remain fixed upon his. After a few moments Richton harrumphs and continues toward the opposite rectangular table, Dad in tow.

"Jerk," Sarah whispers in my ear.

Nodding, I turn toward Sarah. "Bully," I whisper back.

I turn back toward Richton, and he is directing Dad's wife, Florence, to sit on their left, behind their table. Florence sits, and I watch as she looks up and across the courtroom. She does not look at me either.

Dad and Richton are the only ones in the courtroom still standing. The two are at their table, appearing confident, almost at ease. They whisper back and forth as Dad turns around, scanning the courtroom. Checking his watch, he smiles. I watch the two men continue their exchange and see Dad turn around again, scan the courtroom, and then check his watch.

"Who's he looking for? There's no one here except Matt and Florence," I whisper to Sarah.

"Does he have any witnesses coming?" Sarah asks, shrugging.

"Not that I know of," I whisper. "We have three on our list, but Olivia's in the hospital. I know Margaret and Tom are here, so we're good. Why is he smiling? See? He's looking back again."

A harbinger of change revealed itself in the form of a subtle, squeaking hinge. The back courtroom doors opened, and my attorney entered with Tom Kearny and Margaret Foster behind her. They took their seats on my side of the courtroom.

I sigh and look at my father. His mouth begins twitching as the color drains from his face. He turns away from Margaret and Tom and, looking down now, places both of his palms on the table, as if to steady himself.

I wonder if he will look like this when he meets God.

His head still hanging, he tilts his ear toward Richton, now whispering intently. After a moment, Richton clears his throat quietly, his boisterous demeanor muted.

Our attorney approaches our table.

"So," she whispers to both of us, a look of relief on her face. "Richton and your dad were convinced our witnesses wouldn't follow through. They were so convincing, even I was wondering."

"Why would he think that?" Sarah asks.

"He was talking about some kind of loyalty, friendship or something? I guess they all went to the same church for a long time?"

The judge enters the courtroom and our attorney stops talk-ing. The bailiff announces the judge's name and we all rise. The judge reads off the case number and glances toward Dad.

Richton makes a motion to forgo the testimony of any witnesses in exchange for a compromise, of course taking into consideration my father's fixed income and limited retirement.

"What is the defendant prepared to offer?" asks the judge.

"One thousand dollars," says Richton.

Our attorney speaks up. "This is quite a surprise, Your Honor. I met with counsel prior, and there was no willingness to negotiate. May I also remind Your Honor that the mediation panel awarded each of my clients one hundred thousand dollars. Sir, may I have a moment to consult with my clients?"

The judge nods.

"I'd like a meeting with Dad," I whisper.

Sarah nods. "He can give us that. Liz, does he even have one hundred thousand dollars?"

"I don't think so, but he has some retirement property he bought when he retired about seven years ago. I know it's on Diamond Lake in White Cloud, not our old cabin, a new place, near his sis-ter. Could we get the deed to that?" I whisper.

My attorney shares our request then asks how much my father paid for his retirement land. Ten years ago, he paid twenty-five thousand dollars for the property.

After a brief negotiation, it is agreed that Dad will accept full financial responsibility for all court costs as well as an additional one thousand dollars. As we requested, Dad is to conference with us after the proceedings. Last, Dad is ordered to hand over the deed to his lakefront retirement property in White Cloud, Michigan.

As the gavel thumps on the judge's desk, Sarah and I look back at Matt. We are all smiling.

Ushered by a court officer to a small conference room, I grab Matt's hand and he squeezes it.

Florence has already managed to seat herself outside the conference room door.

"How can you—" she begins.

We continue walking without a backward glance, and our attorney closes the door before Florence can finish her sentence.

Inside the conference room Dad and his attorney sit on one side of the table, the side nearest the back wall. I take my seat across from Dad while Matt sits to my right and across from Richton. Sarah stands on my left, leaning against the wall and staring at Dad. Our attorney stands on Matt's right, also leaning against the wall.

"Lizzie and Sarah, I can't believe you think I'm that horrible," my father begins in a bitter, angry tone.

"Stop," I said, holding up my index finger. "This is our meeting, not yours."

Dad folds his arms across his chest, angrily pursing his lips and shaking his head.

"I want you to know that everyone here knows you sexually abused us and you knew what you were doing every time. You tricked us. You used God against us. And I don't *think* you're that horrible; I *know* you're that horrible."

I pause.

"Sarah?" I ask.

In a trembling but clear voice Sarah spoke. "What Liz said was right. You tricked us all along, all us kids. And, it just breaks my heart because"—she takes a deep breath and finishes her sentence in a near whisper—"because you were our father."

A powerful silence fills the room.

"You both know I was on medication and don't remember—"

"Do you happen to know the name of that medication?" Matt interrupts, leaning forward with one palm spread wide open on the table.

My father does not answer.

"Because we should contact the FDA about medicine that makes men sexually abuse little children," Matt concludes.

"I'm just saying, I don't remember—"

"That's a lie," I say boldly. "You do remember."

He shakes his head back and forth.

"Go on and shake your head a thousand times. Go ahead and say 'I don't remember' a thousand times. It will never make it the truth."

I look at Sarah. Tears are still in her eyes.

"Are we done here?" I ask.

She nods her head. We rise and leave the small conference room with Dad and Richton still seated.

* * *

On the way home we went out for dinner and discussed what to do with Dad's retirement property. Selling the land for a substantial amount of money would compromise what we knew to be our motives. We didn't want to give Dad, Todd, or anyone on Dad's side of the family the idea that we were in this for the money.

Using the computer and a calculator, we estimated the appraised value of the property to be around at least fifty thousand dollars.

In order to preserve the spirit and clarity of truth, we decided to sell it for much less.

There was one aunt on my father's side of the family who believed Dad was guilty of molesting his children. She and her husband were on a fixed income. When we called and asked if they would be interested in the property, they expressed their surprise. Indeed they were interested, but they didn't want to offend us by offering what they could afford.

We negotiated briefly, agreeing to sell her the lakefront property for a bargain price: one thousand dollars. No one could questions our motives now.

It was truly the deal of a lifetime.

FORTY-EIGHT

The Pink Chair

It has been a little over six months since the conclusion of the court case.

When I first started therapy, I saw Maureen once a week. Over time I graduated to every other week, then every third week, and now, it's once a month.

In the beginning, I wanted to learn how to take care of myself when I was afraid, and now I am able to do that. Now I'm wondering if I'm strong enough to stop seeing her altogether.

"How will I know it's safe to stop seeing you?" I ask.

Maureen hardly pauses, as if she's been waiting for me to ask the question.

"There are markers that will help you know when you're ready."

"Markers?"

264

"Your list of things to talk about may be shorter. Or the issues you bring up may feel less intense. You may find yourself thinking more about the future than the 'right now.'"

I consider. My lists *have* been shorter. I've often thought on my way to her office that we're going to finish early.

"Matt and I are thinking of moving to Colorado to be near Sarah. Now that the court case is finished, I feel like my work in Michigan is done."

As I say this, I realize I'm saying my work with Maureen is done. We both smile for a moment.

We agree to meet once more, and she suggests lunch at a local restaurant.

* * *

I arrive at the restaurant knowing I am saying goodbye to someone to whom I owe my sanity, my marriage…indeed, my life. How do I tell her this?

We sit down at the restaurant, and Maureen hands me an ivory-colored envelope. I open it, and inside is a card, a gesture that touches me deeply. I know that in the future when I say goodbye to a friend, I will get her a card. I smile at the lovely pink chair on the front of the card.

Dear Liz,

You have somehow found a way in the past five years to find yourself. I am happy for you.

I want to thank you for the honor to know you and the opportunity to share in your rebirth. You are an intelligent, courageous, sensitive woman.

It has been an honor to know you.

Best wishes always,

Maureen

I wonder if she knows the honor has also been mine.

Our lunch is mingled with conversation that feels *different*. She talks about visiting her children over the summer. I share that Matt and I have resigned from our jobs, and in two weeks we'll be living in Colorado.

Shifting in my wooden chair, I realize I have never spoken to Maureen outside of my pink chair.

I realize the pink chair was mine only as long as I needed it.

Like my white wall.

Like Maureen.

After we finish lunch, there is a quiet moment, and Maureen smiles. Her napkin is on the table.

"Are we ready?" she asks.

Nodding, I rise, and she follows suit. We exit the restaurant, the sun at its zenith. The door closes behind us slowly.

It is now fully closed.

I reach out to hug Maureen, and she reciprocates.

"All the best to you, Liz," she says.

"And you," I reply, smiling through my tears.

We release, and she chuckles. "Do you have any other big adventures planned? I mean in addition to picking up and moving to Colorado to start a new life with Matt?" she asks.

"Not that I know of," I reply, also smiling. "We're going to take a few weeks to take in some sights before we start looking for work again."

I wave at her and walk about ten steps toward my car. I hesitate, then turn back toward her.

"You know what, though?" I announce to her from across the parking lot. "I may just write a book."

A f t e r w o r d

Liz is one of many clients I have been lucky to know—people I have looked forward to seeing in spite of dealing with such painful experiences. Many share Liz's courageous spirit, so evident when time after time she would reveal memories that brought her deep, yet undeserved shame. Often, revealing such memories in a safe place with a safe person, shrinks the grip that trauma can have on survivors.

Those who avoid therapy may not realize how much energy is spent on fearing the past and running from it. It is often doing the kind of work Liz describes here that heals. It needs to be at a pace that survivors can choose and have control over, in their own time and in their way.

I let clients know that therapy involves working together as a team: Liz is the expert about herself and her experiences. I have expertise in healing. I needed help in understanding her, and I would help her using what I'd learned over the years. She became an expert on working as a team. Like many clients, she would share the day-to-day, but also difficult information and feelings—a lot involving shame. Shame looms large for survivors, since they are the ones blamed for the abuse. They learn to blame themselves, especially when it happens early in their lives. Liz was gutsy, bringing in experiences that were painful to talk about; but somehow she knew what she needed to do.

It helped that she'd often feel better afterward. Sometimes the overwhelming fear was broken by the cleansing power of getting it out in a safe place with a safe person. It is often my biggest responsibility to provide both.

I take notes and give clients a copy after each session. In addition, Liz took her own notes during our work and often added to them at home. The result was reams of information to draw from to recount our work. While it would be impossible for the dialogue in the sessions to be exact, it is true to the essence of our work.

Liz's book is a blessing to me, and I am so honored by it. A therapist can never participate in the "take your child to work" days. Her memoir allows my family to know a great deal more about my work—work that is a passion for me and a blessing in my life.

It is heartening to see Liz today, with her love for her family and her energy for life. She has always had an indefatigable spirit. It is wonderful to see her rise out of so many years of brutality. I hope her healing can move many of the millions of struggling survivors to believe in the possibility of their own healing.

Maureen McNamara, LMSW, DCSW

Made in the USA
Lexington, KY
05 February 2015